Infectious Diseases Case Studies

Third Edition

A Compilation of 76 Clinical Studies

C. GLENN COBBS, M.D.
Professor of Medicine
Director, Division of Infectious Diseases

FRANK M. GRIFFIN, JR., M.D.
Associate Professor of Medicine

C. KIRK AVENT, M.D.
Associate Professor of Medicine

WILLIAM E. DISMUKES, M.D.
Professor of Medicine

School of Medicine, Division of Infectious Diseases
University of Alabama in Birmingham

Medical Examination Publishing Co., Inc.
an Excerpta Medica company

MEDICAL EXAMINATION PUBLISHING CO., INC.
an Excerpta Medica company
969 Stewart Avenue
Garden City, New York

Library of Congress Card Number
80-27594

ISBN 0-87488-011-4

March 1981

Printed in the United States of America

notice

The editor(s) and/or author(s) and the publisher of this book have made every effort to ensure that all therapeutic modalities that are recommended are in accordance with accepted standards at the time of publication.

The drugs specified within this book may not have specific approval by the Food and Drug Administration in regard to the indications and dosages that are recommended by the editor(s) and/or author(s). The manufacturer's package insert is the best source of current prescribing information.

CONTENTS

INTRODUCTION

This book is intended as a teaching aid for students of infectious diseases, whether those students be residents or seasoned practitioners. We hope that some of the fun we had preparing this manuscript transmits to those who read it. If examination of these cases results in any new knowledge, all the better.

The case studies describe patients seen, for the most part, since the preparation of the second edition. A few of the original case studies have been updated. We hope the patients described are representative of the kind of disorders seen by physicians and students interested in infectious diseases. With only a few exceptions each patient was seen personally at the University of Alabama School of Medicine by at least one of the authors. Reproductions of Gram-stained specimens have been omitted because color reproduction was not feasible. Instead, the findings are described in the text. (It is, of course, critically important for physicians who care for patients with "infectious disease" disorders to examine *personally* preparations of pathological material.) Several questions follow each presentation and the correct answers are indicated along with a brief discussion of points suggested by the case or by the questions.

The answer to the first question that follows a case is often revealed by subsequent questions so, for the most fun, the reader is advised to try not to peek ahead.

Following the answers a few references are cited. For the most part, sections in medical textbooks have not been cited as references. It should be obvious that the standard texts generally contain excellent, well-organized discussions of most infectious disease subjects. The journal references cited are intended to complement the texts.

Since the cases are drawn from an inpatient consultative service, the more serious infectious disease disorders are emphasized. Outpatient problems and pediatric infectious diseases have not been stressed.

There may be occasions where the opinions expressed in this book differ from those of some authorities. We hope that some of the fun of reading these cases will result from identification of these areas of disagreement. It is likely that unless the reader is stimulated sufficiently to track down additional information for himself he'll not learn much. One minor point:

unless stated to the contrary, all patients may be assumed to have no history of penicillin allergy.

We wish to thank the Medical Examination Publishing Company for supporting this project. We also wish to thank Ms. Susan Lamb for her assistance and patience in the preparation of this manuscript.

C. Glenn Cobbs, M.D.
Frank M. Griffin, Jr., M.D.
C. Kirk Avent, M.D.
William E. Dismukes, M.D.

INFECTIOUS DISEASES

CASE 1

HISTORY

This 31-year-old man was transferred to University Hospital in July because of fever which was unresponsive to antimicrobial agents. He had been well until 10 days previously when he noted the onset of myalgias, low grade fever and abdominal pain. These symptoms persisted until 6 days prior to admission when, following a softball game, he felt weak and noted more fever and headache. Five days prior to admission he saw his private physician who admitted him to a local hospital where he was treated with ampicillin, gentamicin and carbenicillin. In spite of this treatment his fever persisted as did his weakness and he was transferred. The patient had no history of recent travel nor ingestion of unusual foods. No one else in his immediate family had been sick. There were a dog and a cat at home. The patient related several insect bites during the last few weeks prior to onset of his illness.

EXAMINATION

Temperature was 104°F, respiration 26 per minute, pulse 110, blood pressure 95/70. There was mild pharyngeal erythema but no nuchal rigidity. The spleen was palpable and there was a diffuse macular erythematous rash over the abdomen and lower back, along with petechiae on the dorsum of both feet, around the ankles and right forearm.

LABORATORY DATA

Admission laboratory work revealed anemia, leucopenia and marked thrombocytopenia, (platelet count 5000). The serum LDH was 700 IU per deciliter, the SGOT was 173 IU, the CPK was 2000 IU. Otherwise the admitting laboratory work was unremarkable. Weil-Felix results, at the time of admission, OX-19, OX-2, and OX-K, all 0.

QUESTIONS

1. WHICH OF THE FOLLOWING DIAGNOSTIC AND THERAPEUTIC MANEUVERS SHOULD BE CARRIED OUT IMMEDIATELY?
   A. Blood culture
   B. Bone marrow biopsy and culture
   C. Liver spleen scan
   D. Splenic aspiration and culture
   E. Lumbar puncture
   F. Treatment for Rocky Mountain spotted fever

2. WHICH OF THE FOLLOWING STATEMENTS ABOUT ROCKY MOUNTAIN SPOTTED FEVER IS/ARE CORRECT?
   A. Therapy of Rocky Mountain spotted fever should await serologic confirmation of the illness
   B. Most patients with Rocky Mountain spotted fever are inhabitants of the western United States
   C. Severe headache is a common accompaniment of this disorder
   D. The rash of Rocky Mountain spotted fever generally begins on the trunk and spreads to the extremities
   E. A history of tick bite may be elicited in more than half the patients with Rocky Mountain spotted fever
   F. It may be transferrable by blood

Coincident with parenteral chloramphenicol therapy and supportive measures the patient's temperature lysed and he generally improved. A serum obtained 8 days after admission revealed a proteus OX-19 titer of greater than 1:160, OX-2 and OX-K still O.

3. WHICH OF THE FOLLOWING STATEMENTS REGARDING THE DIAGNOSIS OF ROCKY MOUNTAIN SPOTTED FEVER IS/ARE CORRECT?
   A. The Weil-Felix test is positive in the vast majority of patients at the time of hospital admission
   B. The etiologic rickettsia may be recovered from tissue

C. An immunofluorescent test for ricksettial antigen in tissue offers a potentially rapid diagnostic tool
D. The most common misdiagnosis in children is measles or atypical measles

ANSWERS

1. (A, F) Sudden onset of a febrile illness during the summer months in the southeast United States should always alert the physician to the possibility of Rocky Mountain spotted fever. In addition the failure of the disorder to respond to penicillin type agents further supports that diagnosis. While there could be a variety of other disorders responsible for this patient's illness it is prudent to begin therapy for Rocky Mountain spotted fever at the time of admission. Blood cultures should be obtained in any patient with fever and undiagnosed illness, but a bone marrow biopsy, liver spleen scan and splenic aspiration are inappropriate. Lumbar puncture would probably not be indicated either early on.

2. (C, E, F) Prior to 1930 all cases of Rocky Mountain spotted fever had been reported from the western United States but since that time the southeastern part of the country has been the site of the vast majority of patients with this disorder. The two principle vectors in the United States are Dermacentor andersoni, the wood tick, which is prevalent in the Rocky Mountain states, and Dermacentor variabilis, the dog tick which is the vector in the southeastern United States. As mentioned above therapy for Rocky Mountain spotted fever should not be delayed while waiting for a positive Weil-Felix test. Headache is a very common symptom in patients with this disease. The rash classically begins on the ankles and wrists, is erythematous and macular and subsequently may become petechial and spread to the trunk. A history of tick bite may be elicited from as many as 85% of patients with this disorder. The report by Wells et al, describes a patient who developed RMSF six days after transfusion with a unit of blood collected from a donor who was incubating that disease.

3. (B, C, D) Antibody directed against the antigens of the proteus X organism (OX-19, OX-2, OX-K) are often not present at the time of admission of a patient with this disorder. Techniques for direct isolation of rickettsia from tissue are available but are dangerous and have lead to severe and even fatal illness in laboratory workers. Therefore they should not be attempted except in a research setting. In contrast the examination of tissue for rickettsia or rickettsial antigen by means of the immunofluorescent test is promising but also not available routinely

yet. Measles is probably the most common misdiagnosis in children with RMSF.

REFERENCES

1. Woodward WE, Hornick RB. Rickettsia ricketsii (Rocky Mountain Spotted Fever). In: Mandell GL, Douglas RG Jr., and Bennett JE, eds. Principles and Practices of Infectious Diseases. New York: John Wiley & Sons, 1979; 1508-14.

2. Hattwick MAW, O'Brien RJ, Hanson, BF. Rocky Mountain spotted fever: Epidemiology of an increasing problem. Ann Intern Med 1976; 84:732.

3. Johnson JE, Kadull PJ. Rocky Mountain spotted fever acquired in a laboratory. New Engl J Med 1967; 277:842.

4. Fleisher G, Lennette ET, Honig P. Diagnosis of Rocky Mountain spotted fever by immunofluorescent identification of Rickettsia rickettsii in skin biopsy tissue. J Pediatrics 1979; 95:63.

5. Wells GM, Woodward TE, Fiset, P, Hornick RB. Rocky Mountain spotted fever caused by blood transfusion. J Am Med Assn 1978; 239:2763.

6. Philip RN, Casper EA, MacCormack JN, et al. A comparison of serologic methods for diagnosing of Rocky Mountain spotted fever. Am J Epidemiol 1977; 105:56.

7. Oster CN. Early diagnosis of Rocky Mountain spotted fever. Arch Int Med 1979; 139:400.

CASE 2

HISTORY

A six-year-old boy is hospitalized because of fever and disorientation. He had spent the previous night in a sleeping bag on the floor of his grandparents' house. He awakened the morning of admission feeling well, but within two hours, he began to complain of malaise, headache, and discomfort over the right anterior chest. At that time, his mother noted a small ulcer with an area of surrounding erythema on the anterior chest. Over the next few hours, the area became more painful and the anterior chest became markedly swollen and developed a brawny discoloration.

EXAMINATION

On physical examination at the time of admission, approximately 8 hours after the first symptom, the patient is acutely ill and delirious with a temperature of 105°F. There is a 4 mm shallow ulcer just above the right nipple with a 2 cm area of surrounding erythema. The entire anterior chest is edematous with a brawny discoloration.

LABORATORY DATA

The white blood cell count is 16,000 with a marked left shift; the hematocrit is 25%. The urine is burgundy colored with 4+ hemoglobin; no red cells, white cells or casts are seen in the sediment. Lumbar puncture is normal. Gram's stain of an aspirate of the subcutaneous area reveals a few polymorphonuclear leukocytes; no bacteria are seen. Chest roentgenogram is normal; specifically, no gas is seen in the soft tissues.

QUESTIONS

1. THE MOST LIKELY CAUSE OF THE PATIENT'S ILLNESS IS
   - A. group A streptococcus
   - B. *Staphylococcus aureus*
   - C. black widow spider toxin
   - D. brown recluse spider toxin
   - E. *Clostridium perfringens*
   - F. *Yersinia pestis*
   - G. *Francisella tularensis*
   - H. *Hemophilus influenzae*
   - I. *Rickettsia rickettsii* (the cause of Rocky Mountain spotted fever)

2. WHICH OF THE FOLLOWING STATEMENTS IS/ARE TRUE?

A. Bites of the brown recluse spider are usually quite painful
B. Plague is not acquired in the United States
C. Tularemia may be transmitted to man by tick bite
D. At the bedside, hemoglobinuria may be distinguished from myoglobinuria by centrifuging plasma and examining the supernate for pink discoloration
E. Administration of calcium is useful in treating complications of brown recluse spider bites

ANSWERS

1. (D) The lesion of the anterior chest was an insect bite. The chief question at the time of initial evaluation was whether the bite had become infected and bacteria were responsible for the clinical picture or whether a toxin injected by the insect was responsible. The patient had massive necrosis and ischemia of the tissues of the chest wall and massive hemolytic anemia; his entire illness can be accounted for by the toxin of the brown recluse spider. Clostridium perfringens elaborates a hemolytic toxin and could cause a similar clinical picture. However, the absence of microbial forms on Gram's stain of tissue juice and the inability to detect gas in tissues by either physical examination or roentgenogram argue strongly against clostridial infection. The other bacteria listed may cause hemolysis only as a part of the picture of disseminated intravascular coagulation; they do not do so directly.

2. (C, D) The initial bite of the brown recluse spider is typically painless; the site may become painful later, as tissue ischemia develops. Plague is endemic in the southwestern United States. The urine dipstick measures both hemoglobin and myoglobin as hemoglobin. A useful test to distinguish myoglobinuria from hemoglobinuria is performed by centrifuging blood and observing the color of the supernatant plasma. Myoglobin is a small molecule which is rapidly filtered by the glomerulus; therefore, the concentration in plasma, even in patients with severe myoglobinuria, is usually sufficiently low that plasma will not be discolored. Because hemoglobin is a larger molecule, and therefore filtered less rapidly, plasma of patients with hemoglobinuria is nearly always pink. Calcium is recommended for the treatment of black widow spider bites; it is not effective for treating complications of brown recluse spider bites. Optimal therapy of brown recluse spider bites and their complications is not well defined. See the first three references below for a more detailed discussion of the topic.

REFERENCES

1. Majeski JA, Durst GG, Jr. Necrotic arachnidism. South Med J 1976; 69:887.

2. Perry WJ. The brown recluse spider in Alabama: A report of five cases. J Med Assn State Ala 1975; 44:552

3. Auer AI, Hershey FB. Surgery for necrotic bites of the brown spider. Arch Surg 1974; 108:612.

4. Vorse H, Seccareccio P, Woodruff K, Humphrey GB. Disseminated intravascular coagulopathy following fatal brown spider bite. J Ped 1972; 80:1035.

5. Berger RS. The unremarkable brown recluse spider bite. J Am Med Assn 1973; 225:1109.

6. von Reyn CF, Weber NS, Tempest B, et al. Epidemiologic and clinical features of an outbreak of bubonic plague in New Mexico. J Infect Dis 1977; 136:489.

7. Boyce JM. Recent trends in the epidemiology of tularemia in the United States. J Infect Dis 1975; 131:197.

CASE 3

HISTORY

A 60-year-old white male was admitted to University Hospital because of fever and abdominal pain. Six months previously the patient had noted a skin rash. After brief treatment by his local physician he was referred to a dermatologist who made a diagnosis of exfoliative dermatitis and initiated corticosteroid therapy. Approximately 40 mg prednisone daily were required to control the process. One week prior to admission the patient noted the onset of fever, abdominal pain and diarrhea, and because of this was admitted to the hospital.

EXAMINATION

On physical examination the patient appeared seriously ill with fever of 103°F. The rash was present and there was mild abdominal pain.

LABORATORY DATA

Laboratory examination was unremarkable. On the second hospital day the patient's diarrhea became worse as did the abdominal pain. Surgery consultants were called in but did not feel there was a clear indication for laparotomy. On the fifth hospital day the patient became more toxic, febrile, hypotensive and died.

QUESTIONS

1. WHICH OF THE FOLLOWING SHOULD HAVE BEEN CONSIDERED IN THE DIFFERENTIAL DIAGNOSIS OF THIS PATIENT'S ILLNESS?
   - A. Acute appendicitis
   - B. Mesenteric vein thrombosis
   - C. Disseminated Strongyloides stercoralis infestation
   - D. Pseudomembranous colitis
   - E. Candida colitis

At post mortem examination, larval forms consistent with strongyloides were found invading deep into bowel wall and a few worms were demonstrated in lung tissue. In addition blood cultures obtained on the day prior to death were positive for Klebsiella pneumoniae.

2. WHICH OF THE FOLLOWING STATEMENT REGARDING STRONGYLOIDES STERCORALIS IS/ARE CORRECT?

A. In addition to the usual life cycle which involves man and soil, strongyloides may complete its life cycle entirely in the human or entirely in the soil
B. Strongyloides infection in man is most easily diagnosed by finding the characteristic eggs in a stool specimen
C. Strongyloides infection may be suspected by the occurrence of cross-reacting complement fixing antibodies to filarial antigens
D. Strongyloides is acquired by ingestion of the infectious eggs
E. Rash may occur at some time after initial infection in patients with strongyloides infestation

3. WHICH OF THE FOLLOWING STATEMENTS ABOUT THE STRONGYLOIDES HYPER-INFESTATION SYNDROME IS/ARE TRUE?

A. Eosinophilia is characteristic
B. Most patients with strongyloides infection have underlying acquired or congenital disorders of host defenses
C. Involvement of renal parenchyma is especially common when hyper-infestation occurs
D. Many patients with strongyloides infection have concomitant gram-negative bacillary bacteremia caused by Klebsiella
E. The antimicrobial agent of choice is thiabendazole
F. The larval form may be seen in sputum in this syndrome

ANSWERS

1. (C)

2. (A, C, E) While the usual life cycle of Strongyloides stercoralis involves invasion of skin by filariform larvae, transportation to the lung, reproduction in the small intestine, and excretion of the rhabditiform larva in stool, the life cycle may occur completely in the host, so called auto-infection, or completely in the soil, the so called indirect cycle. Diagnosis from stool examination is made by observing the rhabditiform larva; eggs are rarely seen in stool. Complement fixing antibodies to filarial antigens are present in approximately 75% of patients with strongyloides infestation. An erythematous urticarial skin eruption may occur in patients with strongyloides infection at some time after their initial encounter with the parasite.

3. (B, D, E, F) While eosinophilia is quite common in patients with strongyloides infestation of the intestine, it is often absent in patients with the hyperinfection syndrome. On occasion this is due to andecedent corticosteroid therapy which antedated extraintestinal invasion. Hyperinfection has been reported almost exclusively in patients with some variety of host defense disorder. Lung and central nervous system are common extraintestinal sites of invasion. The kidney is almost never involved. Gram-negative bacteremia has been reported in a significant number of patients with this disorder. It is possible that injury to the bowel by the parasite facilitates transmucosal invasion by bacteria. Thiabendazole is the appropriate agent for treatment of all varieties of strongyloides disease. The larval form is occasionally seen in sputum of patients with this syndrome.

REFERENCES

1. Purtilo DT, Meyers WM, Connor DH. Fatal strongyloidiasis in immunosuppressed patients. Am J Med 1974; 56:488.

2. Kanani SR, Rees PH. The diagnosis of strongyloidiasis with special reference to the value of the filarial complement fixation test as a screening test. Trans R Soc Trop Med Hyg 1970; 64:246.

CASE 4

HISTORY

A 74-year-old white, diabetic man is admitted to the hospital because of fever and lower abdominal pain. He has a history of recurrent urethral strictures and perineal fistulae complicating gonorrhea acquired and treated many years ago. Over the past 4 days he has had chills and fever and a progressively painful and swollen perineum.

EXAMINATION

On physical examination his temperature is 103.6°F, his blood pressure is 110/62, and his pulse is 118 and thready. A cellulitis with foul purulent drainage involves his perineum and scrotum. His sclerae are icteric.

LABORATORY DATA

His hematocrit is 27% and his WBC count is 14,900 with a shift to the left. His bilirubin is 4 mgm/dl and the SGOT and alkaline phosphatase are normal.

QUESTIONS

1. CORRECT MANAGEMENT SHOULD INCLUDE
   A. volume expansion with IV fluids
   B. x-ray films of the involved area
   C. antibiotics
   D. surgical drainage

2. APPROPRIATE ANTIBIOTIC REGIMENS INCLUDE
   A. cefazolin and gentamicin
   B. penicillin and gentamicin
   C. clindamycin and gentamicin
   D. chloramphenicol and gentamicin

Wide surgical drainage is accomplished. On the third hospital day the patient is still critically ill. Blood cultures drawn on admission are growing an anaerobic gram-negative bacillus, later identified as <u>Bacteroides fragilis</u>.

3. WHICH OF THE FOLLOWING STATEMENTS IS/ARE TRUE?
   A. Necrotizing suppuration of the perineum (Fournier's gangrene) is usually associated with <u>B. fragilis</u>
   B. The hyperbilirubinemia is caused by <u>Bacteroides</u>

C. Most Bacteroides fragilis are sensitive to clindamycin, chloramphenicol, carbenicillin, and metronidazole
D. Bacteroides fragilis is the likely single pathogen causing this patient's infection

ANSWERS

1. (A, B, C, D) X-ray films are done to determine the presence and extent of gas formation.

2. (C, D) Coverage must include antibiotics effective against anaerobes as well as other enteric organisms. Cephalosporins are, in general, poor agents for anaerobic infections. Bacteriodes fragilis is penicillin resistant.

3. (A, B, C) Hyperbilirubinemia occurs in half of patients with Bacteroides bacteremia; the mechanism is not known. Most cases of Fournier's gangrene are polymicrobial in etiology.

REFERENCES

1. Chow AW, Guze LB. Bacteroidaceae bacteremia: Clinical experience with 112 patients. Medicine (Baltimore) 1974; 53:93.

2. Finegold SM, Bartlett JG, Chow AW, et al. Management of anaerobic infections. Ann Intern Med 1975; 83:375.

3. Finegold SM. Therapy for infections due to anaerobic bacteria. An overview. J Infect Dis (Suppl) 1977:525.

4. Fischer JR, Conway MJ, Takeshita RT, Sandoval MR. Necrotizing fasciitis. J Am Med Assn 1979; 241:803.

CASE 5

HISTORY

A 42-year-old alcoholic man was transferred to the Birmingham Veterans Administration Hospital for management of pneumonia. He was well until six days previously when he noted the onset of fever and abdominal pain. Five days before transfer he was admitted to a local hospital where he received supportive therapy for presumed pancreatitis. Two days before transfer the abdominal pain improved but fever persisted and a left lower lobe infiltrate was noted on the repeat chest roentgenogram. Because of the progressive pneumonia, hypoxia and confusion, he was transferred to the Veterans Hospital.

EXAMINATION

On physical examination he was delirious and appeared icteric. Blood pressure was normal; his respiratory rate was 48, temperature was 103°F. There was dullness to percussion and rales over the left lower lobe.

LABORATORY DATA

His laboratory examination revealed a white count of 6400 with a left shift, SGOT of 300, bilirubin 4.0 mgm%, 2+ proteinuria and arterial hypoxemia. The chest roentgenogram confirmed the presence of a left lower lobe infiltrate. Sputum examination revealed numerous polymorphonuclear leukocytes and scant bacterial flora.

QUESTIONS

1. WHICH OF THE FOLLOWING DISORDERS IS MOST LIKELY?
   - A. _Mycoplasma pneumoniae_ pneumonia
   - B. _Staphylococcus aureus_ pneumonia
   - C. Primary influenza pneumonia
   - D. Legionnaires' disease
   - E. Q fever

Despite broad spectrum antimicrobial agents and supportive care in the intensive care unit, the pulmonary infiltrate progressed to involve the right lung as well and the patient died on the 10th hospital day. Examination of post mortem lung tissue demonstrated the agent of Legionnaires' disease.

2. WHICH OF THE FOLLOWING IS/ARE TRUE REGARDING LEGIONNAIRES' DISEASE?
   - A. The causative agent is a pleomorphic faintly gram-negative bacillus for which the name _Legionella pneumophila_ has been proposed

B. The agent can be easily cultured from a "good" expectorated sputum specimen
C. Penicillin G appears to be the antimicrobial agent of choice in treatment of patients with Legionnaires' disease
D. Proteinuria and abnormal liver function may be observed in patients with Legionnaires' disease
E. There appears to be an association of the Legionnaires' disease agent and air conditioning cooling towers

3. WHICH OF THE FOLLOWING IS/ARE ACCEPTABLE METHODS FOR ESTABLISHMENT OF A DIAGNOSIS OF LEGIONNAIRES' DISEASE?
A. Culture of trachael aspirate, bronchial washing, pleural fluid or lung tissue on nutrient agar supplemented with iron and cyteine
B. Direct fluorescent antibody examination of tracheal aspirate, bronchial washings, pleural fluid or lung tissue
C. Indirect fluorescent antibody determinations on acute and convalescent sera

ANSWERS

1. (D) The combination of progressive pneumonia with gastrointestinal symptoms, accompanied by evidence of hepatic injury, confusion and proteinuria should suggest the possibility of Legionnaires' disease. Pneumonia caused by other bacteria can certainly not be excluded early on. This clinical picture is not typical of primary influenza pneumonia which typically follows a day or two of influenza symptoms and then rapidly progresses to bilateral alveolitis. Q fever may cause atypical pneumonia syndrome and liver involvement may occur; therefore, that diagnosis is possible.

2. (A, D, E) The Legionnaires' disease microorganism is a slowly-growing, strictly aerobic, gram-negative bacillus. It stains weakly by Gram's method and better with the Gimenez stain. Gas-liquid chromatographic studies have shown that the organism contains large amounts of branched-class fatty acids, unlike any gram-negative bacillus previously studied. It can be cultured on artificial media supplemented with cysteine and ferric salts but recovery is only feasible when a relatively uncontaminated specimen is available. Routine expectorated sputum with numerous mouth bacteria present is not a good specimen since the Legionnaires' disease organism will be obscured by more rapidly proliferating bacteria. The total American experience, gained in the laboratory and in actual outbreaks, supports the use of erythromycin as the agent

of choice in the treatment of Legionnaires' disease. Laboratory evaluations, including agar dilution susceptibility tests, prophylaxis of infection in embryonated eggs, and protection studies in guinea pigs, have shown that erythromycin and rifampin are the two most effective antimicrobial agents against Legionella. Laboratory abnormalities noted in patients with Legionnaires' disease have included a mild to moderate leukocytosis with a predominance of polymorphonuclear cells, elevated liver enzymes, hyponatremia, hypophosphatemia, proteinuria, and microscopic hematuria. Several epidemiologic investigations suggest that exposure to dusty conditions or air conditioning cooling towers may be important in the pathogenesis of Legionnaires' disease.

3. (A, B, C) Culture of an appropriate specimen, direct fluorescent antibody examination of tissue and indirect fluorescent antibody of acute and convalescent sera are all appropriate methods of substantiating the diagnosis of Legionnaires' disease.

REFERENCES

1. Fraser DW, Tsai TR, Orenstein W, et al. Legionnaires' disease. Description of an epidemic of pneumonia. N Engl J Med 1977; 297:1189.

2. McDade JE, Shepard CC, Fraser DW, et al. Legionnaires' disease. Isolation of a bacterium and demonstration of its role in other respiratory disease. N Engl J Med 1977; 297:1197.

3. Alexander WJ, Dismukes WE. Legionnaires' disease: Review of the clinical disease, causative organism, and epidemiology. South Med J 1979; 72:1174.

4. Broome CV, Fraser DW. Epidemiologic aspects of Legionellosis. Epidemiologic Reviews 1979; 1:1.

CASE 6

HISTORY

A 6-year-old girl developed low grade fever, malaise and a vesicular eruption typical of varicella. She is brought to the hospital six days after the onset of the illness because of somnolence.

EXAMINATION

Physical examination reveals a lethargic child with a temperature of 101°F. The general physical examination is normal and there are no focal neurologic signs. Nuchal rigidity is not present. She has resolving crusted lesions typical of varicella.

LABORATORY DATA

Initial laboratory data are unremarkable except for abnormal liver function studies.

QUESTIONS

1. LUMBAR PUNCTURE WOULD MOST LIKELY REVEAL
   A. 200 white cells, chiefly lymphocytes; protein of 85; normal glucose
   B. no white cells; protein of 85; normal glucose
   C. no white cells; protein of 35; normal glucose
   D. 200 white cells, chiefly lymphocytes; protein of 85; glucose of 15
   E. 2000 white cells, chiefly neutrophils; protein 85; glucose of 15

2. IN ADDITION TO VARICELLA, WHICH ONE OF THE FOLLOWING IS MOST FREQUENTLY ASSOCIATED WITH REYE'S SYNDROME?
   A. Influenza A
   B. Influenza B
   C. Parainfluenza virus
   D. Respiratory syncytial virus
   E. Adenovirus
   F. Rhinovirus

3. WHICH OF THE FOLLOWING IS/ARE TRUE?
   A. Reye's syndrome can be characterized as post-viral encephalitis
   B. Influenza B generally occurs in pandemics, as does influenza A
   C. The serous fluid in vesicles of varicella lesions is only minimally infectious
   D. Parainfluenza virus is the most common cause of croup

E. A respiratory syncytial virus vaccine is efficacious in preventing or attenuating the course of respiratory syncytial virus bronchiolitis in young children

ANSWERS

1. (C) While the patient could have varicella encephalitis, it is statistically much more likely that she has Reye's syndrome, in which case the cerebrospinal fluid will be normal.

2. (B)

3. (D) Reye's syndrome is a post-infectious disorder of uncertain etiology. It is characterized by abnormal mitochondrial function of hepatocytes and neurons, leading to hepatic insufficiency and encephalopathy but not encephalitis. Influenza A occurs in pandemics; influenza B is an endemic disease. The vesicular fluid in varicella is highly infectious. A killed respiratory syncytial virus vaccine was developed and used for several years. Far from being efficacious, however, its use resulted in severe, often fatal, pulmonary disease when immunized children were later infected with RS virus. Needless to say, it is not currently used.

REFERENCES

1. Schiff GM. Reye's syndrome. Ann Rev Med 1976; 27:447.

2. Corey L, Rubin RJ, Hattwick MAW. Reye's syndrome: Clinical progression and evaluation of therapy. Pediatrics 1977; 60:708.

3. Cramblett HG. Croup (epiglottitis, laryngitis, laryngotracheobronchitis). In: Kendig EL Jr, Chernik V. Disorders of the Respiratory Tract in Children, Third Edition. Philadelphia: WB Saunders Co, 1977:353-60.

4. Euler LV, Kantor FS, Hsiung GD. Studies of parainfluenza viruses. 1. Clinical, pathological and virological observations. Yale J Biol Med 1963; 35:523.

5. Chanock RM, Kapikian AZ, Mills J. Influence of immunological factors in respiratory syncytial virus disease of the lower respiratory tract. Arch Environ Health 1970; 21:347.

CASE 7

HISTORY

This was the first University Hospital admission for this 70-year-old black male who was brought to the emergency room by his family because of confusion and disorientation of one day's duration. The patient had been in relatively good health until the morning of admission when his neighbors failed to observe him take his usual morning walk. They went to his house where he was found lying on the floor confused and disoriented.

EXAMINATION

On physical examination at the emergency room, his vital signs were unremarkable except for temperature of 103°F. Inspection revealed a thin, confused black male, who was agitated and restless. The general physical examination was unremarkable. The neurologic examination revealed he was oriented to person but not to time or place. He appeared agitated and there were seemingly purposeless movements of both upper extremities. Grasp reflexes were present bilaterally and there was a Babinski sign noted on the left. The sensory examination was unremarkable. Lumbar puncture revealed a low opening pressure.

LABORATORY DATA

The cerebrospinal fluid contained 17 white cells per mm^3, 90% were mononuclear. The CSF glucose was 54 mgm % and the protein was 113 mgm %.

QUESTIONS

1. THIS ILLNESS IS MOST CONSISTENT WITH
   - A. aseptic meningitis
   - B. meningococcal bacteremia and meningitis
   - C. encephalitis
   - D. brain abscess
   - E. chronic subdural hematoma

2. WHICH OF THE FOLLOWING STATEMENTS CONCERNING ST. LOUIS ENCEPHALITIS IS/ARE TRUE?
   - A. The etiologic agent is a Togavirus
   - B. Most patients infected with St. Louis encephalitis virus exhibit clinical symptoms and signs
   - C. Severity of clinical disease is approximately proportional to patient age; children are usually less severely affected than adults

D. Aseptic meningitis, caused by SLE agent, is more common in younger individuals than in older ones
E. The etiologic virus is easily recovered from blood and spinal fluid of patients with disease
F. Tremor, suggesting basal ganglia involvement, is a common clinical finding in patients with SLE

3. WHICH OF THE FOLLOWING STATEMENTS REGARDING THE EPIDEMIOLOGY OF ST. LOUIS ENCEPHALITIS IS/ARE CORRECT?
A. Horses are the major reservoir in nature
B. Control measures are most effective when directed primarily against mosquitoes
C. There appear to be two epidemiologic varieties of St. Louis encephalitis
D. Chickens may be utilized as sentinel birds for surveillance

ANSWERS

1. (C) This clinical summary describes a patient with St. Louis encephalitis.

2. (A, C, D, F) Arboviruses are enveloped RNA agents with a spherical nucleocapsid and icosahedral symmetry. Classification is somewhat complex. Presently, arboviruses are divided into the togaviruses, bunyaviruses, and orbiviruses. The agent responsible for St. Louis encephalitis falls into the Group B togavirus category designated flaviviruses. During urban epidemics of St. Louis encephalitis, the vast majority of infected patients remained asymptomatic. The ratio of clinically ill to asymptomatic infected patients is in the order of 1:100. The severity of clinical illness with St. Louis encephalitis is proportional to patient age. Aseptic meningitis seems to be more common in younger patients with St. Louis encephalitis than in older ones where encephalitis is most common. It is difficult to recover the St. Louis encephalitis viral agent from spinal fluid or blood. Tremor is common in St. Louis encephalitis, presumably because of basal ganglia involvement.

3. (B, C, D) Birds, not horses, are the main reservoir in nature for the virus of St. Louis encephalitis. The agent is spread by mosquitoes, usually Culex tarsalis, Culex papiens and Culex quinquefasciatus. There appear to be two epidemiologic types of illnesses; urban, occurring in cycles, and endemic rural disease.

REFERENCE

1. Luby JP, Sulkin SE, Sanford JP. The epidemiology of St. Louis encephalitis: A Review. Ann Rev Med 1969; 20:329.

CASE 8

HISTORY

A 35-year-old woman is hospitalized because of fever, wheezing and cough. She was in good health until two months earlier when she began to experience episodic fever, mild wheezing, dyspnea and non-productive cough. For the past month, she has noted daily wheezing and dyspnea, which have progressively worsened, and has had fever to 102°F.

EXAMINATION

Physical examination reveals a mildly ill appearing woman who coughs frequently during the interview. Examination of the chest reveals generalized expiratory wheezes and patches of medium and fine inspiratory rales in the left upper lung field and over the right and left lung bases. The remainder of the physical examination is normal.

LABORATORY DATA

Laboratory evaluation reveals a white blood cell count of 14,000 with 20% eosinophils. Branching septate mycelial forms are seen in a wet preparation of the sputum. Chest roentgenogram reveals generalized hyperaeration of the lung fields with patchy infiltrates in the right lower lobe, left lower lobe and left upper lobe. Culture of the sputum reveals *Aspergillus fumigatus*.

QUESTIONS

1. WHICH OF THE FOLLOWING WOULD YOU EXPECT IN THIS PATIENT?
   - A. Elevated serum IgE level
   - B. Depressed serum IgA level
   - C. Immediate hypersensitivity to aspergillus antigens by skin testing
   - D. Serum precipitins to aspergillus antigens
   - E. Invasion of the lung parenchyma with aspergillus on lung biopsy

2. APPROPRIATE THERAPY INCLUDES WHICH OF THE FOLLOWING?
   - A. Administration of corticosteroids
   - B. Administration of amphotericin B intravenously
   - C. Administration of amphotericin B by inhalation
   - D. Administration of nystatin by inhalation
   - E. Administration of penicillin

3. WHICH OF THE FOLLOWING CONDITIONS IS/ARE ASSOCIATED WITH THE PULMONARY INFILTRATE AND EOSINOPHILIA (P. I. E.) SYNDROME?

A. Allergy to nitrofurantoins
B. Ascariasis
C. Strongyloidiasis
D. Sarcoidosis
E. Toxoplasmosis
F. Enterobiasis (pinworm)

4. WHICH OF THE FOLLOWING STATEMENTS IS/ARE TRUE?

A. The development of peripheral eosinophilia appears to depend upon a product elaborated by T lymphocytes
B. Eosinophilia is a feature of Addison's disease
C. Eosinophils elaborate large quantities of the vasoactive materials histamine and SRS-A
D. The function of eosinophils in allergy is dependent upon the eosinophils' surface receptors for IgE
E. Eosinophils are capable of phagocytizing and killing many bacteria, but not so efficiently as are polymorphonuclear neutrophils
F. Aspergillus rarely causes invasive disease except in immunosuppressed patients
G. One role of eosinophils appears to be to act in concert with antibodies to destroy some helminth larvae

ANSWERS

1. (A, C, D) The patient has allergic pulmonary aspergillosis a disorder initiated by inhalation of aspergillus spores with endobronchial proliferation of the fungus. The symptoms are caused by a type I allergic reaction to antigens of the mold, and, while pulmonary infiltrates are the rule, they are composed only of inflammatory exudate. The yeast does not invade lung tissue in this syndrome.

2. (A) Treatment consists of removing the patient from the source of aspergillus spores, often found in dirty air-conditioning equipment, and treating acute episodes with corticosteroids. Anti-fungal therapy is not required.

3. (A, B, C, D) Causes of the P. I. E. syndrome include allergic reactions to certain drugs, certain vasculitides, the pulmonary migratory phases of invasive helminths, allergic reactions to inhaled antigens, eosinophilic leukemia, and certain forms of the hypereosinophilic syndrome. Protozoa, such as <u>Toxoplasma gondii</u>, do not cause eosinophilia. Pinworm is strictly an

intestinal parasite; it has no larval migration phase and therefore is not a cause of the P. I. E. syndrome.

4. (A, B, E, F, G) Basophils and mast cells, not eosinophils, elaborate large quantities of histamine and SRS-A. The function of basophils and mast cells, not of eosinophils, is dependent upon the presence of IgE receptors on their surfaces. If eosinophils play a unique role in host defense, it is likely to be destruction of vasoactive substances elaborated by mast cells. It seems most unlikely that they are uniquely equipped to efficiently phagocytize or kill microorganisms or even to destroy helminthic parasites, although they are able to perform both these functions.

REFERENCES

1. Golbert TM, Patterson R. Pulmonary allergic aspergillosis. Ann Intern Med 1970; 72:395.

2. Patterson R, Fink JN, Pruzansky JJ, et al. Serum immunoglobulin levels in pulmonary allergic aspergillosis and certain other lung diseases, with special reference to immunoglobulin E. Am J Med 1973; 54:16.

3. Rosenberg M, Patterson R, Mintzer R, et al. Clinical and immunologic criteria for the diagnosis of allergic bronchopulmonary aspergillosis. Ann Intern Med 1977; 86:405.

4. Young RC, Bennett JE, Vogel CL, et al. Aspergillosis. The spectrum of the disease in 98 patients. Medicine 1970; 49:147.

5. Adickman M, Tuthill TM. Pulmonary infiltrates and eosinophilia. Postgrad Med 1976; 60:143.

6. Liebow AA, Carrington CB. The eosinophilic pneumonias. Medicine 1969; 48:251.

7. Basten A, Boyer MH, Beeson PB. Mechanism of eosinophilia. II. Role of the lymphocyte. J Exp Med 1970; 131:1288.

8. Wasserman SI, Goetzl EJ, Austen KF. Inactivation of slow reacting substance of anaphylaxis by human eosinophil arylsulfatase. J Immunol 1975; 114:645.

9. Cline MJ. Microbicidal activity of human eosinophils. J Reticuloendothel Soc 1972; 12:332.

10. Butterworth AE, David JR, Franks D, et al. Antibody-dependent eosinophil-mediated damage to ^{51}Cr-labeled *Schistosoma mansoni*: Damage by purified eosinophils. J Exp Med 1977; 145:136.

CASE 9

HISTORY

A 72-year-old white man was admitted because of pneumonia. He had smoked for many years and had mild dyspnea on exertion. Five days prior to admission he noted the onset of cough productive of yellow-green sputum. One day prior to admission, because of fever and worsening cough, his family suggested he seek medical advice.

EXAMINATION

On physical examination findings were consistent with right lower lobe pneumonia. Gramed stained smear of a "good" sputum specimen revealed numerous polymorphonuclear leukocytes and many small pleomorphic gram-negative bacilli.

QUESTIONS

1. THE DIFFERENTIAL DIAGNOSIS OF THIS PATIENT'S ILLNESS SHOULD INCLUDE
   A. influenza virus pneumonia
   B. pneumonia caused by *Mycoplasma pneumoniae*
   C. *Haemophilus influenzae* pneumonia
   D. pneumococcal pneumonia
   E. staphylococcal pneumonia
   F. Legionnaires' disease

2. WHICH OF THE FOLLOWING ANTIMICROBIAL AGENTS IS/ARE APPROPRIATE FOR AN ADULT WITH SUSPECTED *HAEMOPHILUS INFLUENZAE* PNEUMONIA?
   A. Penicillin G
   B. Tetracycline
   C. Ampicillin
   D. Chloramphenicol
   E. Vancomycin

The *Haemophilus influenzae* strain was resistent to ampicillin by disc susceptibility testing.

3. WHICH OF THE FOLLOWING STATEMENTS REGARDING AMPICILLIN RESISTANT *HAEMOPHILUS INFLUENZAE* IS/ARE TRUE?
   A. Most strains of ampicillin resistant *Haemophilus influenzae* belong to serotype B.
   B. Ampicillin resistance among *Haemophilus influenzae* strains is due to beta lactamase production by the microorganism

C. Kirby-Bauer disc susceptibility testing is sufficient for delineation of ampicillin resistant strains
D. No strains of Haemophilus influenzae have been reported which have been resistant to chloramphenicol
E. Many older patients with proven Haemophilus influenzae disease have demonstrable defects in the complement system

ANSWERS

1. (C) All of the other options are less likely. Influenza virus pneumonia is typically associated with bilateral diffuse alveolitis, severe toxicity and hypoxemia, and a sputum containing polymorphonuclear leukocytes, but few if any identifiable microorganisms. Mycoplasma pneumoniae usually does not cause lobar pneumonia and a dominant bacterium would not be expected on Gram stain. The Gram stain is also not suggestive of a pneumococcal or staphylococcal etiology. Legionnaires' disease may present in this fashion, but the etiologic microorganism is not identifiable by Gram staining technique.

2. (C, D) While some strains of Haemophilus influenzae are resistant to ampicillin, this is sufficiently uncommon so that ampicillin is still appropriate as initial therapy for most patients with suspected haemophilus disease as long as there is no central nervous system involvement. In the latter case, chloramphenicol should be included in initial therapy.

3. (A, B, E) Ampicillin resistance is most common among serotype B strains of Haemophilus influenzae. This resistance is mediated by penicillinase production coded for by a plasmid. Kirby-Bauer disc susceptibility testing is not sufficient for precise delineation of ampicillin resistance among Haemophilus influenzae; direct determination of penicillinase production by the bacteria is a superior method. A rare strain of Haemophilus influenzae has been reported to be resistant to chloramphenicol. Older patients with Haemophilus influenzae disease, which may include such disorders as pneumonia, septic arthritis and bacteremia occasionally have demonstrable defects in the complement system.

REFERENCES

1. Levin DC, Schwarz MI, Matthay RA, et al. Bacteremic Hemophilus influenzae pneumonia in adults. A report of 24 cases and a review of the literature. Am J Med 1977; 62:219.

2. Slack MPE, Wheldon DB, Turk DC. A rapid test for beta-lactamase production by *Haemophilus influenzae*. Lancet 1977; 2:906.

CASE 10

HISTORY

A 42-year-old man is hospitalized because of fever, sore throat and disorientation. He was well until one week earlier when he developed sore throat and fever to 101°F. He treated himself with salicylates and throat lozenges. However, his throat became progressively worse, such that by the day of admission, he was unable to swallow.

EXAMINATION

Physical examination reveals a toxic, confused man with marked swelling of the left side of the jaw, neck and upper chest wall. His temperature is 105°F. Examination of the mouth and pharynx reveals erythema of the left tonsil and peritonsillar area, a fluctuant left peritonsillar mass, and marked deviation of the uvula to the right. The soft tissues of the jaw, neck and upper chest are erythematous and indurated with pitting edema. There is no evidence of jugular vein thrombophlebitis. The remainder of the physical examination is normal.

LABORATORY DATA

The white blood cell count is 17,000 with a marked left shift. Urinalysis is normal. Lumbar puncture is normal. Blood cultures are obtained and plans are made for drainage of the fluctuant mass.

QUESTIONS

1. THE MICROORGANISMS WHICH ARE MOST LIKELY TO CAUSE SUCH AN ILLNESS INCLUDE
   - A. group A streptococcus
   - B. *Pseudomonas aeruginosa*
   - C. *Corynebacterium diphtheriae*
   - D. *Staphylococcus aureus*
   - E. *Neisseria gonorrheae*
   - F. mouth anaerobes
   - G. *Hemophilus influenzae*

2. WHICH OF THE FOLLOWING STATEMENTS IS/ARE TRUE?
   - A. Ludwig's angina is an infection of the floor of the mouth which usually follows dental abscess
   - B. The presence of jugular vein thrombophlebitis and jaundice in a patient with parapharyngeal infection should

lead one to suspect Staphylococcus aureus as the most likely offending microorganism

C. Patients with cellulitis of the face who develop bilateral proptosis and complete extraocular muscle palsy should be anticoagulated

D. The bacterium which most commonly causes parotitis is group A streptococcus

E. The antimicrobial agent of choice for the initial treatment of bacterial sinusitis in adults is ampicillin

3. ISOLATION OF WHICH OF THE FOLLOWING BACTERIA FROM THE THROAT OF A PREVIOUSLY HEALTHY PATIENT WHO HAS DEVELOPED PHARYNGITIS REQUIRES ANTIMICROBIAL THERAPY?

A. Staphylococcus aureus
B. Group A streptococcus
C. Corynebacterium diphtheriae
D. Neisseria gonorrheae
E. Escherichia coli
F. Pseudomonas aeruginosa
G. Neisseria meningitidis
H. Mycoplasma pneumoniae
I. Streptococcus pneumoniae
J. Yersinia pestis
K. Mycobacterium fortuitum
L. Candida albicans
M. Actinomyces israeli

ANSWERS

1. (A, D, F) The patient has a peritonsillar abscess with complicating cellulitis of the neck and chest wall. He probably also has bacteremia. Peritonsillar abscess is an unusual complication of pharyngitis. While the cause of the initial pharyngitis is often group A streptococcus, peritonsillar abscess may be caused either by group A streptococcus, Staphylococcus aureus, or mouth anaerobes.

2. (A, E) When jugular vein thrombosis complicates parapharyngeal infection, one should be especially suspicious that anaerobes, especially bacteroides species, are involved. While it is somewhat controversial, most authorities would not recommend anticoagulation for cavernous sinus thrombosis because the cerebral infarction resulting from venous occlusion is often hemorrhagic. Staphylococcus aureus causes the vast majority of cases of bacterial parotitis. In adults, pneumococcus and Hemophilus influenzae are responsible for the majority of cases of sinusitis; therefore, ampicillin is an appropriate initial antimicrobial agent.

3. (B, C, D, J) The other microorganisms listed do not usually cause pharyngitis, but do colonize the throat of man with varying degrees of frequency.

REFERENCES

1. Levitt GW. Cervical fascia and deep neck infections. Otolaryngol Clin N Amer 1976; 9:703.

2. Bartlett JG, Gorbach SL. Anaerobic infections of the head and neck. Otolaryngol Clin N Amer 1976; 9:655.

3. Mead RH III. Peritonsillar and parapharyngeal infections. New Engl J Med 1978; 298:894.

4. Meyers BR, Lawson W, Hirschman SZ. Ludwig's angina. Case report, with review of bacteriology and current therapy. Am J Med 1972; 53:257.

5. Goldberg MH, Harrigan WF. Acute suppurative parotitis. Oral Surg 1965; 20:281.

6. Hamory BH, Sande MA, Sydnor A Jr, et al. Etiology and antimicrobial therapy of acute maxillary sinusitis. J Infect Dis 1979; 139:197.

CASE 11

HISTORY

This was the first University Hospital admission for this 63-year-old black female who was brought to the emergency room on Christmas day by her daughter because she was not "functioning". The patient had been well until eight weeks previously when her daughter noted a gradually progressive loss of memory and decreased appetite. The patient had taken a trip to Michigan six weeks prior to admission and, on returning two weeks later, was noted by her daughter to have severe memory loss and also mild difficulty walking. She was seen by a private physician who admitted her to a local hospital with a presumptive diagnosis of anxiety neurosis. During the next week in the hospital she became progressively mute and tremulous. She was given electric shock treatment without improvement. One week prior to transfer to University Hospital she was noted to have myoclonic jerking, and an EEG showed generalized slow wave activity without localizing signs.

EXAMINATION

The admission physical examination was unremarkable except for the neurologic portion which revealed an alert appearing but mute patient who did not follow commands. Cranial nerves were unremarkable. Clonus was present in the left upper extremity and there was moderate hypertonicity of all four extremities. The tendon reflexes were normal and there was no Babinski sign. The laboratory examination was unremarkable, including a lumbar puncture. During the first three weeks of her hospitalization the patient's neurologic status gradually deteriorated and marked myoclonic jerking and frontal lobe release signs appeared.

QUESTIONS

1. THIS ILLNESS IS MOST SUGGESTIVE OF
   - A. chronic lymphocytic meningitis
   - B. encephalitis caused by an arbovirus agent, for example St. Louis encephalitis.
   - C. Creutzfeldt-Jacob disease
   - D. brain abscess
   - E. myxedema madness

Five weeks after admission to University Hospital, the patient died. At post mortem examination findings characteristic of Creutzfeldt-Jacob disease were found with degeneration and disappearance of nerve cells and astroglial proliferation involving cerebral cortex and basal ganglia.

2. WHICH OF THE FOLLOWING STATEMENTS REGARDING CREUTZFELDT-JACOB DISEASE IS/ARE TRUE?

A. It is considered a slow virus disease
B. It can be transmitted from man to animal and possibly from man to man
C. The agent responsible for Creutzfeldt-Jacob disease is quite resistent to some routine sterilization procedures

3. WHICH OF THE FOLLOWING IS PRESENTLY CONSIDERED A SLOW VIRUS DISEASE IN MAN?

A. Hallevorden-Spatz disease
B. Progressive rubella encephalitis
C. Progressive multifocal leukoencephalopathy
D. Kuru
E. Subacute sclerosing panencephalitis

ANSWERS

1. (C) This steadily progressive myoclonic dementia is typical of Creutzfeldt-Jacob disease. The normal spinal fluid examination essentially rules out chronic lymphocytic meningitis. The time of year and the steady progression of the disorder argues against arbovirus encephalitis, although early on in the patient's course that might be a reasonable possibility. Absence of focal signs and fever and the normal lumbar puncture are somewhat against brain abscess. Myxedema is always a consideration in patients with dementia, but no other typical physical findings were described.

2. (A, B, C) Scrapie of sheep, transmissible mink encephalopathy, Kuru, and Creutzfeldt-Jacob disease are classified in the subacute spongiform encephalopathies and are believed caused by slow virus infection. There are several reports of transmission of Creutzfeldt-Jacob disease from man-to-animal and man-to-man, the latter occuring in one instance via a corneal transplant and in another via silver electrodes which had been sterilized with 70% alcohol and formaldehyde vapor. The latter occurrence suggests the agent is resistant to some sterilization procedures.

3. (B, C, D, E) Progressive rubella encephalitis is associated with congenital rubella infection and results in a child who may appear normal at birth but who later experiences language delay, ataxia, myoclonic jerking, and mental deterioration. It is associated with elevated spinal fluid immunoglobulins and a peculiar granular vasculitis on brain biopsy. Progressive multifocal leukoencephalopathy is a disorder of older patients with males predominating. Usually there is underlying altered

cellular immunity. It produces demyelinating lesions and eosinophilic intranuclear inclusions and clinically there is evidence of diffuse cerebral disease with hemiparesis, visual difficulties, speech changes and a fatal outcome in three to four months. A polyomavirus has been incriminated. Kuru, originally described in the Fore tribe of New Guniea, is a progressive dementia with tremor and is pathologically similar to Creutzfeldt-Jacob disease. It has been transmitted from man to primates. S. S. P. E. is a disorder of children and is thought to be due to chronic rubeola virus infection. Clinically it is characterized by mental deterioration, myoclonus, dystonia and abnormal spinal fluid with elevated protein; on brain biopsy there are type A eosinophilic inclusions. High levels of antibodies to rubeola are found in serum and spinal fluid.

REFERENCES

1. Harter DH. Diseases caused by slow viruses. In: Isselbacher KJ, Adams RD, Braunwald E, Petersdorf RG, Wilson JD. Harrison's Principles of Internal Medicine. New York: McGraw-Hill, 9th Edition. 1980:844-846.

2. Duffy P, Wolf J, Collins G, et al. Possible person-to-person transmission of Creutzfeldt-Jacob disease. N Engl J Med 1974; 290:692.

3. Bernoulli C, Siegfried J, Baumgartner G, et al. Danger of accidental person-to-person transmission of Creutzfeldt-Jacob disease by surgery. Lancet 1977; I:478.

CASE 12

HISTORY

A 68-year-old man with stage IVB Hodgkin's disease is brought to the emergency room because of fever and disorientation. The diagnosis of Hodgkin's disease was made one year earlier at staging laparotomy, at which time the spleen was removed. He had subsequently been doing well on BACOP therapy. His present illness began three days earlier with fever and headache; confusion and disorientation were noted 16 hours prior to admission.

EXAMINATION

Physical examination reveals an acutely ill, febrile, confused man with bilateral Babinski signs. Otherwise, the physical examination is unremarkable.

LABORATORY DATA

The white blood cell count is 10,000 with a normal differential; hematocrit is 38%, platelet count is normal. Urinalysis, liver function tests, and roentgenograms of the skull are normal. Lumbar puncture reveals an opening pressure of 230 mm; 150 leukocytes, of which 65% are lymphocytes, 35% neutrophils; protein of 70; and glucose of 70 with a concomitant serum glucose of 100.

QUESTIONS

1. THERE ARE MANY POSSIBLE CAUSES OF THE PATIENT'S ILLNESS. IF HE HAS ENCEPHALITIS DUE TO TOXOPLASMA GONDII, WHICH OF THE FOLLOWING FINDINGS WOULD YOU EXPECT?
   - A. Intracerebral calcifications visible on skull roentgenogram
   - B. Splenic calcifications visible on abdominal roentgenogram
   - C. Toxoplasma trophozoites in the stool
   - D. Toxoplasma trophozoites visible on a smear of cerebrospinal fluid
   - E. Evidence of healed toxoplasma chorioretinitis
   - F. Serum toxoplasma indirect immunofluorescent antibody titer of 1:256 or greater

2. A PATIENT WHO IS 2 MONTHS PREGNANT IS EVALUATED FOR THE POSSIBILITY OF RECENTLY ACQUIRED TOXOPLASMOSIS. WHICH OF THE FOLLOWING IS/ARE SUFFICIENT TO RECOMMEND THAT SHE HAVE AN ABORTION?

A. History of frequent exposure to the litter box used by her cat, which died three weeks earlier and was found to be excreting oocysts of Toxoplasma gondii.
B. Toxoplasma indirect immunofluorescent antibody titer of 1:256; toxoplasma complement fixation titer negative
C. Toxoplasma indirect immunofluorescent antibody titer of 1:256; toxoplasma complement fixation titer of 1:4
D. Toxoplasma indirect immunofluorescent antibody titer of 1:256, which remains at 1:256 when tested four weeks later; toxoplasma complement fixation titer negative, which remains negative when tested four weeks later.
E. Toxoplasma indirect immunofluorescent antibody titer of 1:256, which remains at 1:256 when tested four weeks later; toxoplasma complement fixation titer, which is negative initially and rises to 1:16 when tested four weeks later

ANSWERS

1. (F) Toxoplasma gondii is an unusual but treatable cause of encephalitis in patients with disorders of delayed hypersensitivity. It is thought to be recrudescence of disease in patients who were initially infected years earlier but who are unable, when delayed hypersensitivity is depressed, to contain the few viable protozoa they have harbored for years. They usually have demonstrable antibody, but do not have intracerebral calcifications or evidence of chorioretinitis, both of which are usually the result of congenital infection. Neither can trophozoites be found in any body fluid. Splenic calcifications are most often the result of healed histoplasmosis, not toxoplasmosis.

2. (E) The decision regarding termination of pregnancy because of the risk of fetal injury from congenital toxoplasmosis is one physicians face frequently. It should be made only after consultation with an expert in the field. The serologic titers of the pregnant woman are critically important in determining whether infection is recent or remote. The IFA titer becomes positive about two weeks after initial infection, rises to 1:several thousand, then remains at a level of about 1:256 - 1:1000 for life. The CF titer becomes positive about 4 weeks after initial infection, rises to about 1:8 - 1:16, then falls to zero over about a year. If one measures these titers serially over about one month, he can usually discern whether infection has occurred

recently or whether a positive IFA represents remote infection. Since only pregnant women who have been recently infected are at risk of infecting the fetus, this distinction is critically important. We re-emphasize that consultation with an expert in the field should be obtained to aid in decisions regarding pregnancy termination.

REFERENCES

1. Krick JA, Remington JS. Toxoplasmosis in the adult - an overview. New Engl J Med 1978; 298:550.

2. Ruskin J, Remington JS. Toxoplasmosis in the compromised host. Ann Intern Med 1976; 84:193.

3. Remington JS, Anderson SE. Diagnosis and treatment of pneumocystosis and toxoplasmosis in the immunosuppressed host. Transplant Proc 1973; 5:1263.

4. Alford CA, Stagno S, Reynolds DW. Congenital toxoplasmosis: Clinical, laboratory and therapeutic considerations, with special reference to subclinical disease. Bull NY Acad Med 1974; 50:211.

5. Rao NA, Font RL. Toxoplasmic retinochoroiditis. Arch Ophthalmol 1977; 95:273.

CASE 13

HISTORY

A 24-year-old male was admitted because of a skin rash and fever. Ten days previously, he was given erythromycin for cough and fever. Five days later he noted the onset of an erythematous rash on his hands. Another physician, suspecting streptococcal cellulitis, prescribed penicillin. During the following three days the rash worsened with extensive erythematous, macular lesions appearing on the extremities. There was also involvement of the lips and mucous membranes of the mouth where large hemorragic bullae were present.

EXAMINATION

On physical examination the patient was seriously ill with extensive skin and mucous membrane eruption having the characteristics of the Stevens-Johnson syndrome.

QUESTIONS

1. WHICH OF THE FOLLOWING HAS/HAVE BEEN SUSPECTED AS AN ETIOLOGY OF THE STEVENS-JOHNSON SYNDROME?
   - A. Drug reaction
   - B. Microbial infectious disease
   - C. Physical agents such as X-ray therapy
   - D. All of the above

2. WHICH OF THE FOLLOWING STATEMENTS CONCERNING DRUG ALLERGY IS/ARE CORRECT?
   - A. Drugs usually produce allergic reactions in man by combining with host macromolecules
   - B. Most drugs must be metabolized in vivo before conjugation with protein can occur
   - C. Anaphylaxis in man is usually mediated by IgM antibodies
   - D. Circulating immune complexes are responsible for the syndrome of serum sickness
   - E. Plasma cells may occasionally be observed in the blood of patients with serum sickness

3. WHICH OF THE FOLLOWING STATEMENTS ABOUT ERYTHROMYCIN IS/ARE CORRECT?
   - A. Erythromycin is an aminoglycoside antimicrobial agent
   - B. Cholestatic hepatitis with eosinophilia has been reported following use of some erythromycin preparations

C. Erythromycin is an acceptable substitute for penicillin G in patients with group A beta hemolytic streptococcal pharyngitis
D. Erythromycin possesses excellent activity against all anaerobic bacteria

ANSWERS

1. (D) Drugs probably account for the majority of instances of Stevens-Johnson syndrome. A review published several years ago suggests there may be three patterns of this disorder. In the first, Stevens-Johnson syndrome occurs in previously well patients without any antecedent drug therapy. In the second group, the disorder follows drug therapy of respiratory or urinary tract symptoms. Finally, Stevens-Johnson syndrome may follow drugs administered for other reasons. The occurrence of the syndrome in the second group of patients suggested to some an infectious etiology.

2. (A, B, D, E) Drug allergy is usually the result of an interaction of the drug or a drug metabolite with serum macromolecules, usually protein. Anaphylaxis is usually mediated by IgE. Serum sickness is a result of circulating immune complexes and their deposition in various sites. Plasma cells may occasionally be found in the circulation of patients with this disorder.

3. (B, C) Erythromycin is a macrolide antibiotic consisting of a large lactone ring to which deoxy sugars are attached. Its mechanism of antimicrobial action appears to involve inhibition of protein synthesis, probably by binding to the 50S subunit of the bacterial ribosome. Erythromycin estolate, the lauryl sulfate salt of the proprionyl ester (Ilosone[R]) causes cholestatic jaundice in some patients. This side effect appears to be much more common in adults and for that reason this particular preparation is probably not justified in that group and the FDA has begun proceedings to remove it from the market. Erythromycin is an acceptable substitute for penicillin for therapy of group A beta hemolytic streptococcal pharyngitis. Some anaerobic bacteria, particularly the anaerobic cocci, are relatively susceptible to erythromycin. Others, such as _Bacteroides fragilis_ and fusobacterium, are not susceptible. For that reason erythromycin is not a good choice for life threatening infectious disease caused by anaerobic bacteria, especially where _Bacteroides fragilis_ may be present.

REFERENCES

1. Bianchine JR, Macaraeg PVJ Jr, Lasagna L, et al. Drugs as etiologic factors in the Stevens-Johnson syndrome. Am J Med 1968; 44:390.

2. Finegold SM. Anaerobic bacteria in human disease. New York: Academic Press. 1977:531.

3. Lyell A, Gordon AM, Dick HM, Sommerville RG. Mycoplasms and erythema multiforme. Lancet 1967; 2:1116.

4. Parker CW. Drug allergy. N Engl J Med 1975; 292:511, 732, 957.

CASE 14

HISTORY

A 65-year-old man presents because of fever and back pain of four weeks' duration.

EXAMINATION

Physical examination reveals a non-ill appearing man with a temperature of 100°F and tenderness over the lower thoracic spine. Neurologic examination is intact.

LABORATORY DATA

Roentgenograms reveal destruction of the T-10, T-11 interspace with partial disintegration of both T10 and T11 vertebral bodies and a paraspinous mass. Intermediate strength PPD is 17 mm. Chest roentgenogram is normal.

QUESTIONS

1. APPROPRIATE INITIAL MANAGEMENT OF THIS PATIENT INCLUDES
   A. drainage of the paraspinous abscess and culture of the material obtained
   B. administration of isoniazid and either ethambutol or rifampin
   C. administration of nafcillin
   D. initially bed rest and subsequently treatment with a back brace
   E. immediate placement of the patient into a spica cast
   F. laminectomy with fusion of the spine

The patient is placed on isoniazid and rifampin and is improved and afebrile four weeks later. Two weeks thereafter, however, he complains of right flank pain and develops fever to 102°F. Serum creatinine is 2.4 mg% (it was normal six weeks earlier).

2. THE MOST LIKELY CAUSE OF THE PATIENT'S CURRENT PROBLEM IS
   A. bacterial pyelonephritis
   B. tuberculous nephritis
   C. isoniazid
   D. rifampin
   E. none of the above

3. WHICH OF THE FOLLOWING STATEMENTS IS/ARE TRUE?
   A. Thrombocytopenia due to rifampin occurs more frequently when rifampin is employed intermittently than when it is employed daily

B. The patient presented most likely acquired *Mycobacterium tuberculosis* infection within the 3 years preceding the onset of his symptoms
C. Optic neuritis is a complication of treatment with isoniazid
D. Optic neuritis is a complication of treatment with ethambutol
E. It is virtually impossible to distinguish radiographically neoplastic vertebral disease from tuberculous spondylitis
F. It is virtually impossible to distinguish radiographically staphylococcal spondylitis from tuberculous spondylitis

ANSWERS

1. (A, B, D) There are two reasonable initial approaches. (1) Have an orthopedic or neurosurgical consultant aspirate material from the paraspinous abscess or biopsy the affected disc. Stain and culture the material for bacteria, mycobacteria, and fungi. If acid fast bacteria are seen or if no diagnosis is made by examination of the smears, begin anti-tuberculous treatment. (2) The clinical picture in combination with a markedly positive PPD skin test make tuberculous spondylitis very, very likely. It is reasonable to treat the patient for tuberculosis and follow the temperature curve and clinical picture without invasive attempts to establish a diagnosis by culture. Treatment of Pott's disease rarely requires either operation or a body cast unless neurologic signs are present.

2. (D) The clinical picture of fever, flank pain, and renal failure is characteristic of rifampin nephrotoxicity, an unusual side effect of rifampin.

3. (A, C, D, F) Most rifampin side effects, including thrombocytopenia, occur more commonly with intermittent therapy than with continuous therapy. While it is impossible to determine when the patient was initially infected with *M. tuberculosis*, epidemiologic studies indicate that most elderly patients who develop tuberculous disease acquired infection many years previously. While optic neuritis more commonly occurs as a result of ethambutol toxicity, INH may also cause it. Infectious spondylitis typically begins in an inter-vertebral disc space then spreads to both adjacent vertebral bodies. Neoplastic vertebral disease, while it may involve multiple vertebral bodies, usually involves each individually, begins near the center of the vertebral body, and only very late in the course involves intervertebral disc spaces.

REFERENCES

1. Davidson PT, Horowitz I. Skeletal tuberculosis. A review with patient presentations and discussion. Am J Med 1970; 48: 77.

2. Berney S, Goldstein M, Bishko F. Clinical and diagnostic features of tuberculous arthritis. Am J Med 1972; 53:36.

3. Sanders WE. Rifampin. Ann Intern Med 1976; 85:82.

4. Weinstein L. Drugs used in the chemotherapy of tuberculosis and leprosy. In: Goodman LS, Gilman A. The Pharmacological Basis of Therapeutics. New York: Macmillan Co., 1975: 1201-1223.

CASE 15

HISTORY

A 23-year-old female presents to her private physician because of sore throat and a skin rash. She was in excellent health until eight days earlier when she developed sore throat, malaise, chills and fever. She was seen by another physician and given ampicillin capsules. Her constitutional symptoms continued for four or five days, and then began to abate, but the pharyngitis became progressively worse. The day prior to presentation she noted a generalized pruritic erythematous rash.

EXAMINATION

Physical examination reveals a temperature of 100°F. The pharynx is erythematous, and there is a whitish exudate over the tonsils and posterior pharynx. A right submaxillary node is enlarged and tender. The spleen tip is palpable in the LUQ. A generalized maculopapular, erythematous rash is present.

QUESTIONS

1. THE MOST USEFUL DIAGNOSTIC TEST WOULD BE
   A. throat culture
   B. mononucleosis spot test
   C. serial determinations of Coxsackie A-9 complement fixation titers
   D. serial determinations of rubella complement fixation titers
   E. determination of serum levels of IgM antibody to ampicillin

2. STUDIES OF THE EPSTEIN-BARR VIRUS (EBV) AND SERUM ANTIBODIES TO IT HAVE SHOWN WHICH OF THE FOLLOWING TO BE TRUE?
   A. Only those people who have no detectable antibody to EBV appear to be susceptible to infectious mononucleosis
   B. IgG antibodies to viral capsid antigen (VCA) are detectable for only several weeks after infection, and thus are useful in establishing the diagnosis of infectious mononucleosis
   C. EBV has been found in most cases of Burkitt's lymphoma in which virus identification has been attempted
   D. Since antibodies to Epstein-Barr virus nuclear antigen (EBNA) may appear 3 to 4 weeks later than antibodies to VCA, rising titers of anti-EBNA may be more useful in making a serologic diagnosis of infectious mononucleosis

3. WHICH OF THE FOLLOWING IS/ARE TRUE?
   A. A mononucleosis-like syndrome following massive transfusion with fresh blood may be caused by cytomegalovirus
   B. It is unusual to have hepatic involvement in the mononucleosis-like syndrome due to cytomegalovirus
   C. It is unusual to have hepatic involvement in the mononucleosis-like syndrome due to Toxoplasma gondii
   D. Peripheral neuropathy, Guillain-Barre syndrome, and meningitis may be seen in infectious mononucleosis
   E. Nasopharyngeal carcinoma in African and Oriental patients is associated with high titers of antibodies to E-B virus

ANSWERS

1. (B) The clinical disorder described is typical of mononucleosis. Development of a rash following ampicillin has been described in almost 100% of patients with mononucleosis.

2. (A, C, D) Antibodies against EB virus have been demonstrated to appear in virtually all patients with infectious mononucleosis. In contrast to the heterophile antibodies, IgG antibodies to VCA and EBNA persist for life. Anti-VCA antibodies appear at the time of clinical presentation. Since anti-EBNA antibodies are first detectible 3 weeks later, the appearance of anti-EBNA antibodies in a patient who was previously anti-VCA positive and anti-EBNA negative is strong evidence of recent EB virus infection.

3. (A, C, D) The so-called post-perfusion syndrome may be related to infection with cytomegalovirus transmitted by fresh blood. Hepatic involvement is universal in cytomegalovirus infection. Hepatic involvement is very unusual in the mononucleosis-like syndrome caused by Toxoplasma gondii infection in adults.

REFERENCES

1. Epstein MA, Achong BG. Pathogenesis of infectious mononucleosis. Lancet 1977; 2:1270.

2. Horwitz CA, Henle W, Henle G, et al. Clinical evaluation of patients with infectious mononucleosis and development of antibodies to the R-component of the Epstein-Barr virus induced early antigen complex. Am J Med 1975; 58:330.

3. Hewetson JF. The role of Epstein-Barr virus (EBV) in various human disorders. South Med J 1975; 68:1271.

4. Evans AS, Niederman JC, McCollum RW. Seroepidemiologic studies of infectious mononucleosis with EB virus. New Engl J Med 1968; 279:1121.

5. Pullen H, Wright N, Murdock JM. Hypersensitivity reactions to antibacterial drugs in infectious mononucleosis. Lancet 1967; 2:1176.

6. Henle W, Henle G. Epstein-Barr virus and infectious mononucleosis. New Engl J Med 1973; 288:263.

7. Evans AS. Infectious mononucleosis and related syndromes. Am J Med Sci 1978; 276:325.

CASE 16

HISTORY

A 45-year-old chronic alcoholic is hospitalized because of delirium tremens and fever.

EXAMINATION

Physical examination reveals a disoriented, combative man with a temperature of 102°F and tachycardia. Hepatomegaly, ascites and signs of chronic liver disease are unchanged from previous admissions. The remainder of the physical examination is normal.

LABORATORY DATA

The hematocrit is 33%, white blood cell count 12,000 with a left shift. Platelet count is normal, urinalysis is normal. Chest roentgenogram is normal. Flat and upright films of the abdomen are normal except for signs of ascites. Abdominal paracentesis reveals clear yellow fluid with 800 cells, 60% of which are polymorphonuclear leukocytes; glucose is normal; protein is 2 gm%. Gram's stain of the fluid reveals no bacteria. Ascitic fluid, blood, and urine are cultured.

QUESTIONS

1. APPROPRIATE INITIAL THERAPY CONSISTS OF
   - A. no antimicrobial therapy
   - B. ampicillin and gentamicin
   - C. isoniazid and ethambutol
   - D. penicillin
   - E. chloramphenicol and gentamicin

2. WHICH OF THE FOLLOWING STATEMENTS IS/ARE TRUE?
   - A. The microorganism most commonly responsible for spontaneous peritonitis in children with nephrotic syndrome and ascites is Escherichia coli
   - B. The microorganism most commonly responsible for spontaneous peritonitis in alcoholics with ascites is Escherichia coli
   - C. In the case of the patient presented, the next day cultures of ascitic fluid grow Klebsiella species; the patient should have a laparotomy with placement of peritoneal drains
   - D. In patients with peritonitis associated with chronic peritoneal dialysis, the dialysis fluid may be used as a vehicle to deliver aminoglycoside antimicrobial agents systemically.

E. Candida albicans and Staphylococcus aureus are normal inhabitants of the human intestinal tract and consequently are frequent pathogens in peritonitis due to a ruptured viscus
F. Instillation of aminoglycoside antimicrobial agents into the peritoneal cavity is not associated with systemic side effects, for these agents are only minimally absorbed by the peritoneal route
G. Treatment of respiratory paralysis caused by aminoglycoside or polymyxin antimicrobial agents includes administration of calcium and neostigmine

ANSWERS

1. (B) The combination of fever without new focal signs, peripheral leukocytosis, and ascitic fluid containing 800 white blood cells makes spontaneous bacterial peritonitis sufficiently likely that the patient should be treated initially. The microorganism most commonly responsible for this syndrome is E. coli, but pneumococcus and other gram-negative enterics may cause it as well. Until cultural data are available, ampicillin and gentamicin is an appropriate combination.

2. (B, D, G) While E. coli is the bacterium most commonly responsible for spontaneous bacterial peritonitis in alcoholics with ascites, pneumococcus is more commonly isolated from children with nephrotic syndrome and ascites who develop spontaneous bacterial peritonitis. Antimicrobial therapy alone, i. e. without peritoneal drainage, is sufficient therapy for patients with this syndrome. The dialysis fluid of patients undergoing chronic peritoneal dialysis has been effectively used as a vehicle to deliver aminoglycoside antimicrobial agents systemically when treating peritonitis. In these patients, delivery of aminoglycosides via the peritoneal route has the advantage of maintaining a nearly constant blood level of the agent, roughly equivalent to the concentration in the dialysis fluid. While Candida albicans can be isolated from the stool of most people and Staphylococcus aureus from the stool of a substantial minority, both microbes are present in very low titer and, in fact, are rarely responsible for peritonitis. As indicated above, aminoglycoside antibiotics are efficiently absorbed from the peritoneal cavity. Therefore, instillation of high concentrations of these agents, e. g. in an irrigation solution during abdominal surgery, may result in toxic blood levels. Very high blood levels of aminoglycosides or polymyxins may result in respiratory paralysis, which should be treated with respiratory support, calcium, and neostigmine.

REFERENCES

1. Weinstein MP, Iannini PB, Stratton CW, Eickhoff TC. Spontaneous bacterial peritonitis. A review of 28 cases with emphasis on improved survival and factors influencing prognosis. Am J Med 1978; 64:592.

2. Conn HO, Fessel JM. Spontaneous bacterial peritonitis in cirrhosis: variations on a theme. Medicine 1971; 50:161.

3. Kline MM, McCallum RW, Guth PH. The clinical view of ascitic fluid culture and leukocyte count studies in alcoholic cirrhosis. Gastroenterology 1976; 70:408.

4. Smithivas T, Hyams PJ, Matalon R, et al. The use of gentamicin in peritoneal dialysis. I. Pharmacologic results. J Infect Dis 1971; 124:S84.

5. Hyams PJ, Smithivas T, Matalon R, et al. The use of gentamicin in peritoneal dialysis. II. Microbiologic and clinical results. J Infect Dis 1971; 124:S77.

6. Pittinger C, Adamson R. Antibiotic blockade of neuromuscular function. Ann Rev Pharmacol 1972; 12:169.

CASE 17

HISTORY

A 67-year-old man was seen by the Infectious Disease service because of fever and confusion of one day's duration. The patient had been well until six months previously when an evaluation for fever and weight loss revealed acute myelomonocytic leukemia. He received cytosine arabinoside and 6-thioguanine in two separate courses. Because of relapse, he was readmitted for another course of therapy. Three weeks following hospital admission, after completion of cytotoxic therapy, the patient developed profound leukopenia. At this time, fever and confusion occurred.

EXAMINATION

Examination revealed the patient was disoriented and confused with temperature of 104°F and hyperreflexia, but no lateralizing neurologic signs. Lumbar puncture was performed and revealed an elevated opening pressure.

LABORATORY DATA

The spinal fluid contained 75 leukocytes, 60% polymorphonuclear and 40% mononuclear, 200 red blood cells, 300 mgm% protein, and 90 mgm% glucose (concomitant peripheral blood glucose 207). Gram stain of spinal fluid revealed gram-positive bacilli without observable spores.

QUESTIONS

1. WHICH OF THE FOLLOWING STATEMENTS IS/ARE TRUE?
   - A. The absence of spore forms rules out the possibility of a clostridial or bacillus etiology
   - B. Penicillin G administered intravenously in large doses is the appropriate initial therapy for this patient
   - C. The finding of gram-positive bacilli on the Gram stained smear of spinal fluid probably indicates contamination
   - D. Patients with bacillus meningitis commonly have associated bacteremia

The spinal fluid culture revealed <u>Bacillus cereus</u>.

2. WHICH OF THE FOLLOWING STATEMENTS CONCERNING BACILLUS SPECIES IS/ARE TRUE?

A. There appear to be two forms of Bacillus cereus food poisoning
B. Demonstration of Bacillus cereus in the stool of a patient with gastroenteritis is an effective way to document the etiology of the disorder
C. Some species of bacillus may be responsible for allergic pulmonary disease among workers in enzyme industries

3. WHICH OF THE FOLLOWING ANTIMICROBIAL AGENTS IS/ARE EFFECTIVE AGAINST MOST STRAINS OF BACILLUS?

A. Penicillin G
B. Methicillin
C. Chloramphenicol
D. Kanamycin
E. Gentamicin
F. Tetracycline
G. Cephalosporins

ANSWERS

1. (D) Although bacillus and clostridia form spores when environmental conditions are suboptimal, one may not see spores in clinical specimens. Penicillin alone is not the antimicrobial agent of choice in suspected bacillus disease since many strains are resistant. There have been reports of contamination of spinal fluid by killed bacteria, but in the circumstances described here this would be a very dangerous assumption. Generally patients with bacillus meningitis have been found to have associated bacteremia.

2. (A, C) There do appear to be two forms of Bacillus cereus food poisoning caused by at least two enterotoxins. One variety which has been reported most commonly following ingestion of rewarmed Chinese rice is probably caused by preformed enterotoxin and usually occurs within one to six hours after the meal. It is analogous to staphylococcal food poisoning. The other form of Bacillus cereus food poisoning has a longer incubation period and may be related to elaboration of enterotoxins in the GI tract. Gram-positive rods are normally found in feces. Cultivation of bacillus or clostridia from the stool would not be sufficient evidence to incriminate either in the pathogenesis of gastroenteritis. Workers in industries where enzymes are produced by bacteria have been reported to develop allergic bronchopulmonary disease.

3. (C, D, E) The various species of bacillus differ in their susceptibility to the antimicrobial agents listed. Only chloramphenicol and the aminoglycosides are active against most strains of these bacteria. Initial therapy of suspected serious bacillus disease should probably include chloramphenicol.

REFERENCES

1. Farrar WE Jr. Serious infections due to "non-pathogenic" organisms of the genus bacillus. Am J Med 1963; 34:134.

2. Ihde DC, Armstrong D. Clinical spectrum of infection due to bacillus species. Am J Med 1973; 55:839.

3. Pennington JE, Gibbons ND, Strobeck JE, et al. Bacillus species infection in patients with hematologic neoplasia. J Am Med Assn 1976; 235:1473.

4. Terranova W, Blake PA. Bacillus cereus food poisoning. N Engl J Med 1978; 298:143.

5. Coonrod JD, Leadley PJ, Eickhoff TC. Antibiotic susceptibility of Bacillus species. J Inf Dis 1971; 123:102.

CASE 18

HISTORY

A 19-year-old enlisted man presents to sick call in Manilla because of "clap". He had sexual contact with a Philippine woman four days earlier. The day before presentation he noted dysuria and a purulent urethral discharge. He denies prior venereal disease. Physical examination is unremarkable except for a purulent urethral discharge, the Gram's stain of which reveals gram-negative diplococci.

QUESTIONS

1. WHICH OF THE FOLLOWING TREATMENT PROGRAMS WOULD BE ASSOCIATED WITH AN UNACCEPTABLE FAILURE RATE IN THIS TYPE OF PATIENT?
   - A. One injection of 4.8 million units of aqueous procaine penicillin G
   - B. One injection of 4.8 million units of aqueous procaine penicillin G plus 1 gm of probenecid PO, given 30 min before the injection
   - C. Ten gm of tetracycline given orally over 4 days
   - D. Ampicillin, 3.5 gm PO, plus 1 gm of probenecid PO in one dose
   - E. Amoxicillin, 3.0 gm PO, plus 1 gm of probenecid PO in one dose

2. WHICH OF THE FOLLOWING HAS/HAVE BEEN INCRIMINATED IN NONGONOCOCCAL URETHRITIS?
   - A. Ureaplasma
   - B. Chlamydia
   - C. Mycobacterium smegmatis
   - D. Mima polymorpha
   - E. Beta hemolytic streptococci

3. WHICH OF THE FOLLOWING MAY BE COMPLICATIONS OF GENITAL GONORRHEA IN THE FEMALE?
   - A. Perihepatitis (Fitz-Hugh-Curtis syndrome)
   - B. Lung abscess
   - C. Proctitis
   - D. Chronic pyelonephritis
   - E. Endocarditis

The patient is treated with 4.8 million units of aqueous penicillin and 1 gm of probenecid. He returns to clinic 5 days later complaining that his persistent discharge has not improved.

4. THE LIKELY CAUSE OF PERSISTENT SYMPTOMS IS
   A. non-gonococcal urethritis
   B. infection with a penicillinase-producing gonococcus
   C. incorrect dose of penicillin
   D. recidivism

ANSWERS

1. (A, D) During and following the Vietnam war physicians noted a striking increase in the numbers of gonococcal isolates with a slightly higher than usual MIC of penicillin. Infections with these organisms would respond to increased doses of penicillin, however.

2. (A, B) A variety of microorganisms has been incriminated as the cause of this disorder. Chlamydia trachomatis can be isolated from 20-40% of patients with NGN. Ureaplasma urealyticum (formerly called T-strain Mycoplasma), Trichomonas, and Candida are also agents capable of causing NGU.

3. (A, C, E)

4. (B) In 1976 penicillinase-producing Neisseria gonorrhoeae (PPNG) were isolated in 11 countries, chiefly southeast Asia, and some spread of the organism has occurred in the United States. Spectinomycin is the agent of choice for PPNG infection.

REFERENCES

1. Gonorrhea. CDC recommended treatment schedules, 1979. Ann Intern Med 1979; 90:809.

2. Holmes KK, Handsfield HH, Wang SP, et al. Etiology of non-gonococcal urethritis. N Engl J Med 1975; 292:1199.

3. Dans PE. Treatment of gonorrhea and syphilis. Part I - gonorrhea. South Med J 1975; 68:1287.

4. Follow-up on antibiotic resistant Neisseria gonorrhoeae. Morbidity and Mortality Weekly Report 1977; 26:29.

5. McCormack WM, Finland M. Spectinomycin. Ann Intern Med 1976; 84:712.

CASE 19

HISTORY

A 63-year-old woman is hospitalized because of fever of 3 weeks' duration. She has been followed by her cardiologist for 15 years because of mitral stenosis secondary to rheumatic fever and, on daily digoxin, has been asymptomatic except for occasional palpitations. Fever began about three weeks prior to admission and has persisted without the appearance of any other symptoms.

EXAMINATION

Physical examination reveals a non-ill appearing woman with a temperature of 101°F. The pulmonic component of the second heart sound is accentuated and there is a slight right ventricular lift. A 2/6 diastolic rumble and opening snap are heard; the remainder of the examination is normal.

LABORATORY DATA

The white blood cell count is normal; the hematocrit is 33%. Urinalysis is normal. On the second hospital day, four of four blood cultures obtained on the day of admission are growing a gram-positive coccus and treatment is begun with penicillin and gentamicin. The following day, the organism is identified as a streptococcus which is susceptible by disc testing to all agents except clindamycin.

QUESTIONS

1. THE SINGLE MOST IMPORTANT DETERMINATION, WHICH WILL DICTATE THE DOSE AND DURATION OF THERAPY AS WELL AS THE ANTIMICROBIAL AGENTS USED, IS
   - A. whether or not the microorganism grows on eosin-methylene blue agar
   - B. whether or not the organism is hemolytic
   - C. whether or not the organism is a group D streptococcus
   - D. the broth dilution susceptibility of the organism to penicillin G
   - E. the patient's response to the first two weeks of treatment with penicillin and gentamicin

By the third hospital day, the patient is afebrile and asymptomatic while receiving penicillin and streptomycin. The laboratory has the following information: The organism is a group D streptococcus; it grows on eosin-methylene blue agar, is not hemolytic, fails to grow in 6.5% sodium chloride, and is inhibited by 0.05 ug/ml of penicillin G when tested by broth dilution.

2. WHICH OF THE FOLLOWING THERAPEUTIC REGIMENS IS/ARE APPROPRIATE FOR THIS PATIENT'S ILLNESS?
   A. Penicillin and Streptomycin for two weeks followed by penicillin alone for an additional two weeks
   B. Penicillin and Streptomycin for two weeks
   C. Penicillin and gentamicin for six weeks
   D. Penicillin alone for 4 weeks
   E. Penicillin and gentamicin for four weeks

3. WHICH OF THE FOLLOWING STATEMENTS IS/ARE TRUE?
   A. A cephalosporin may be substituted for penicillin in the treatment of endocarditis due to most viridans streptococci
   B. A cephalosporin may be substituted for penicillin in the treatment of enterococcal endocarditis
   C. Vancomycin may be substituted for an aminoglycoside in the treatment of streptococcal endocarditis
   D. Ampicillin is adequate prophylaxis for patients with valvular heart disease who are undergoing cystoscopy
   E. Tetracycline plus gentamicin would be an appropriate therapeutic regimen for the patient presented
   F. The patient presented should have proctoscopy and barium examination of the colon

ANSWERS

1. (D) The key microbiologic determination in treating patients with streptococcal endocarditis is the degree of susceptibility of the microorganism to penicillin. If the minimal inhibitory concentration (MIC) of penicillin is less than 0.2 ug/ml, the patient can be treated "less vigorously" (See discussion of question 2, below) than if the MIC of penicillin is greater. This determination cannot be made by disc susceptibility testing. Choices A, B, and C have to do with certain characteristics which help to establish the identity of the streptococcus. While it is of some use to know whether the organism is a viridans streptococcus, enterococcus, etc., it is not the key question. All enterococci are relatively insensitive to penicillin (MIC greater than 0.2 ug/ml), and endocarditis caused by enterococci requires more prolonged treatment. Most viridans streptococci are quite susceptible and can be treated for a shorter duration. Virtually all patients with streptococcal endocarditis respond quickly to treatment with penicillin and gentamicin,

regardless of the degree of the bacterium's susceptibility to penicillin. Dosage and duration of therapy are dependent upon the microbiologic studies discussed above, not upon the patient's initial response to antimicrobial therapy.

2. (A, B, D) From the above discussion, it is apparent that, even though the isolate is a group D streptococcus, it cannot be an enterococcus because of its exquisite susceptibility to penicillin. That it is not an enterococcus is confirmed by its inability to grow in hypertonic medium (6.5% NaCl). Therefore, it is a non-enterococcal group D streptococcus, such as Streptococcus bovis. The patient need not be treated for 4-6 weeks with both penicillin and gentamicin. Regimens A, B and D are those currently accepted for treatment of endocarditis caused by these isolates.

3. (A, F) Cephalosporins may be used in combination with an aminoglycoside in place of penicillin in the treatment of endocarditis caused by streptococci which are exquisitely susceptible to penicillin (and to cephalosporins) but not in the treatment of endocarditis caused by more resistant isolates such as enterococci. Vancomycin may be substituted for penicillin, not for an aminoglycoside. Most authorities recommend adding an aminoglycoside to ampicillin for prophylaxis of genito-urinary procedures. Bacteriostatic agents such as tetracycline have no role in the treatment of endocarditis. About 40% of patients who develop Streptococcus bovis endocarditis have been found to have an intestinal lesion, usually carcinoma, responsible for the initial bacteremia which led to endocarditis. Therefore, all such patients should have radiographic evaluation of the gastrointestinal tract.

REFERENCES

1. Hook EW, Guerrant RL. Therapy of infective endocarditis. In: Kaye D. Infective Endocarditis. Baltimore: University Park Press, 1975; 167-84.

2. Moellering RC Jr, Watson BK, Kunz LJ. Endocarditis due to group D streptococci. Comparison of disease caused by Streptococcus bovis with that produced by the enterococci. Am J Med 1974; 57:239.

3. Hoppes WL, Lerner PI. Nonenterococcal group-D streptococcal endocarditis caused by Streptococcus bovis. Ann Intern Med 1974; 81:588.

4. Steinberg D, Naggar CZ. Streptococcus bovis endocarditis with carcinoma of the colon.. New Engl J Med 1977; 297:1354.

5. Mandell GL, Kaye D, Levison ME, Hook EW. Enterococcal endocarditis. An analysis of 38 patients observed at the New York Hospital-Cornell Medical Center. Arch Intern Med 1970; 125:258.

6. Rahal JJ Jr, Meyers BR, Weinstein L. Treatment of bacterial endocarditis with cephalothin. New Engl J Med 1968; 279:1305.

7. Hook EW III, Johnson WD. Vancomycin therapy of bacterial endocarditis. Am J Med 1978; 65:411.

CASE 20

HISTORY

This was the first Birmingham Veteran's Administration Hospital admission of this 39-year-old white male who presented because of cough, fever and chest pain. Three weeks prior to admission the patient had a syncopal episode while going to the store with a friend. He was taken to a local hospital emergency room. There he noted one of his front teeth was missing. He was treated briefly and discharged. Two weeks later, he noted the onset of coughing, productive of thick purulent sputum, as well as anorexia, fever, and a "flu-like syndrome". Because of this, he came to the hospital, where, on physical examination, rales and ronchi in the left upper lobe were noted. There was no clubbing.

LABORATORY DATA

Admission laboratory work revealed a white blood cell count of 8,000 with 91% polymorphonuclear leukocytes. Chest x-ray is reproduced in Figure 1.

QUESTIONS

1. THIS PATIENT'S DISEASE MOST LIKELY REPRESENTS
   A. pulmonary tuberculosis
   B. putrid lung abscess
   C. <u>Histoplasma capsulatum</u> chronic pulmonary disease
   D. slowly resolving pneumococcal pneumonia

2. WHICH OF THE FOLLOWING STATEMENTS ABOUT PUTRID LUNG ABSCESS IS/ARE CORRECT?
   A. The microbiology of putrid lung abscess is often similar to that of the normal flora of the mouth
   B. Although poor dental hygiene and conditions favoring aspiration clearly predispose to putrid lung abscess, these conditions are rarely found in patients presenting with this disorder
   C. The basal segments of the right lower lobe are the most common sites of putrid lung abscess
   D. Careful examination and culture of expectorated sputum with special attention to precise identification of anaerobic bacteria is useful in the management of patients with putrid lung abscess

3. WHICH OF THE FOLLOWING STATEMENTS REGARDING MANAGEMENT OF PUTRID LUNG ABSCESS IS/ARE CORRECT?
   A. Bronchoscopy is indicated early on in the management of patients with this disorder

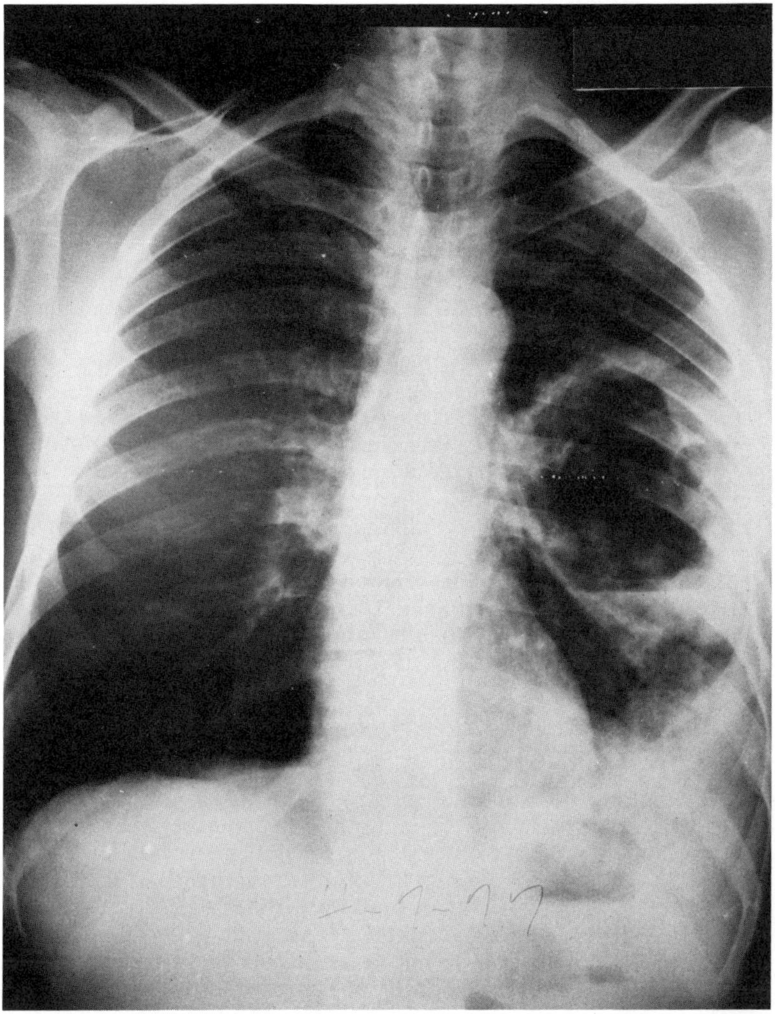

Figure 1

B. Therapy of lung abscess should include antimicrobial agents effective against penicillin-resistant anaerobic bacteria, especially Bacteroides fragilis
C. If an abscess is not resolved by four weeks, surgical resection is necessary
D. Following initial in-hospital evaluation, many patients with putrid lung abscess may be managed as out-patients

ANSWERS

1. (B) This case history and physical examination describe a rather typical patient with putrid lung abscess and, together with the chest roentgenogram, that diagnosis is almost certain.

2. (A) It is natural that the microbial flora of putrid lung abscess should reflect the mouth since aspiration is the antecedent event in most patients. As many as 80% of patients with putrid lung abscess have "oral sepsis" and/or a history of aspiration. The dependent segments of the lung are most susceptible to aspiration induced lung abscess. These include the posterior segment of the right upper lobe and the superior segment of the right lower lobe. Sputum examination and anaerobic culture of material obtained by expectoration will be of no use in therapy of putrid lung abscess since passage through the mouth will contaminate such a specimen and make the results uninterpretable. Sputum obtained by methods which bypass the pharynx such as trans-tracheal aspiration and direct lung puncture will provide more accurate information, but these are potentially dangerous and not usually indicated.

3. (D) There is controversy regarding the precise role for bronchoscopy in management of patients with putrid lung abscess. Generally early bronchostomy is recommended only if the patient remains toxic following an initial trial of antimicrobial therapy, postural drainage and other supportive measures, if the patient is unable to bring up bronchial secretions, or if there is a history of aspiration of solid material, e.g. a tooth. In addition, when there is a likely possibility of tumor or obstructing foreign body, bronchoscopy should be performed. Bronchoscopy is probably not indicated in every patient with putrid lung abscess, especially if the process resolves uneventfully leaving no residua. It is not necessary to treat specifically for resistant anaerobic bacteria such as Bacteroides fragilis. Clinical trials of a number of antimicrobial agents have shown good results when antibiotics were used which did not inhibit or kill that particular microorganism. Penicillin is the drug of choice. Generally, a high dose regimen is employed initially; once the patient has begun to improve, oral

therapy with penicillin or tetracycline is appropriate until the lesion has healed. Resection is unnecessary if there has been complete healing in four weeks. Patients may certainly be treated as outpatients when they have improved sufficiently to leave the hospital.

REFERENCES

1. Bartlett JG, Gorbach SL, Talley FP, Finegold SM. Bacteriology and treatment of primary lung abscess. Am Rev Resp Dis 1974; 109:510.

2. Chidi CC, Mendelsohn HJ. Lung abscess. A study of the results of treatment based on 90 consecutive cases. J Thor and Cardiovas Surg 1974; 68:168.

CASE 21

HISTORY

A 25-year-old male dog catcher was bitten on the hand by a stray dog while attempting to trap the animal. The animal died twelve hours later and the brain was found to contain Negri bodies. The patient had developed serum sickness three years previously after having been treated with antivenom following a rattlesnake bite. He had received a tetanus toxoid booster immunization at that time.

EXAMINATION

Physical examination is normal except for a healing superficial laceration of the right index finger, the site of the dog bite.

QUESTIONS

1. APPROPRIATE PROPHYLAXIS FOR THIS PATIENT CONSISTS OF WHICH OF THE FOLLOWING?
   - A. No treatment necessary
   - B. Administration of horse derived rabies immune globulin and institution of active immunization with rabies vaccine prepared in duck embryos
   - C. Administration of horse derived rabies immune globulin and institution of rabies vaccine prepared in a human diploid cell line
   - D. Administration of human rabies immune globulin and institution of duck embryo vaccine
   - E. Administration of human rabies immune globulin and institution of rabies vaccine prepared in a human diploid cell line
   - F. Administration of tetanus toxoid

2. BITES BY WHICH OF THE FOLLOWING ANIMALS DEMAND PASSIVE AND ACTIVE RABIES PROPHYLAXIS? ASSUME THE ANIMAL CANNOT BE LOCATED.
   - A. Bat
   - B. Squirrel
   - C. Cow
   - D. Fox
   - E. Raccoon
   - F. Skunk
   - G. Rat
   - H. Dog
   - I. Cat

Three days after being bitten by the dog, the patient complains of pain and swelling at the bite site. Examination reveals erythema and tenderness of the area surrounding the wound and slight purulent discharge. Gram's stain of the exudate reveals small gram-negative bacilli.

3. APPROPRIATE INITIAL ANTIMICROBIAL THERAPY WOULD CONSIST OF

A. penicillin
B. cloxicillin
C. gentamicin
D. carbenicillin
E. cephalexin
F. chloramphenicol

ANSWERS

1. (E) The patient needs both active and passive rabies prophylaxis; two varieties of each are available. Immune globulin prepared in horses should no longer be used with the availability of human rabies immune globulin; moreover, the patient has previously experienced serum sickness from horse serum and certainly should not receive it again. A vaccine prepared in a human cell line is available through the CDC. Because of its very limited supply, stringent criteria - known allergy to eggs or ducks, serious reaction to DEV, a bite by an animal known to be rabid, or failure of a series of DEV to elicit sufficiently high antibody titer - are employed for its release. Since the patient has recently received tetanus toxoid, he need not receive it again.

2. (A, D, E, F, H, I) Rodents and cattle almost never carry rabies; therefore, rabies prophylaxis need not be given for bites by these animals. There is a high prevalence of rabies in bats, skunks, racoons, wolves, and foxes, and bites or scratches by any of these animals demand rabies prophylaxis unless the animal is known and the brain can be promptly examined. The only opportunity for discrimination by the physician occurs in the case of a dog or cat bite. If the animal is known and appears healthy, then it can be observed for 10 days, and the patient need not be treated if no signs of rabies develop in the animal. If the animal cannot be located, then the patient should usually receive prophylaxis, although the CDC suggests that the physician may not provide prophylaxis depending upon the circumstances surrounding the bite and the prevalence of domestic animal rabies in the community.

3. (A) The bacterum described is most likely Pasteurella multocida, which is a normal inhabitant of dogs' mouths and a common cause of dog bite infections. It is susceptible to penicillin, and that is the antimicrobial agent of choice.

REFERENCES

1. Public Health Service Advisory Committee on Immunization Practices. Rabies: Risk, management, prophylaxis, and immunization. Ann Intern Med 1977; 86:452.

2. Corey L, Hattwick MAW, Baer GM, Smith JS. Serum neutralizing antibody after rabies postexposure prophylaxis. Ann Intern Med 1976; 85:170.

3. Rubin RH, Sikes K, Gregg MB. Human rabies immune globulin. Clinical trials and effects on serum anti-γ-globulins. J Am Med Assn 1973; 224:871.

4. Fraser DW. Preventing tetanus in patients with wounds. Ann Intern Med 1976; 84:95.

5. Francis DP, Holmes MA, Brandon G. Pasteurella multocida infections after domestic animal bites and scratches. J Am Med Assn 1975; 233:42.

CASE 22

HISTORY

A 57-year-old man was admitted to the Birmingham Veteran's Administration Hospital for chills, fever and sweats of two weeks duration. The patient was well until two weeks previously when he noted sudden onset of hard shaking chills followed by fever and malaise. Chills and fever recurred frequently thereafter with temperature as high as 104°F recorded by the patient. One week prior to admission the patient noted the additional symptom of pain and tenderness in the anterior cervical region.

EXAMINATION

On admission to the hospital, physical examination revealed fever and a mildly enlarged thyroid gland with tenderness, especially in the left lobe. Otherwise the remainder of the physical examination was unremarkable. Routine admission laboratory work was likewise normal.

LABORATORY DATA

Because of tender thyroid gland, thyroid function tests were obtained. The serum T4 was 15 mcg/dl and the serum T3 was 320 ng/dl. A thyroid scan showed markedly decreased uptake at 24 and 48 hours.

QUESTIONS

1. WHICH OF THE FOLLOWING IS THE MOST LIKELY CAUSE OF THE PATIENT'S FEVER?
   - A. Collagen vascular disease involving the thyroid gland
   - B. Pyogenic thyroiditis
   - C. Subacute (deQuervain's) thyroiditis
   - D. Fungal disease of the thyroid gland
   - E. Sarcoid thyroiditis

2. WHICH OF THE FOLLOWING STATEMENTS ABOUT SUBACUTE (DEQUERVAIN'S) THYROIDITIS IS/ARE CORRECT?
   - A. It is probably caused by a virus
   - B. It is an autoimmune disorder
   - C. There is striking association with the HLA-Bw 35 histocompatibility antigen
   - D. Hypothyroidism is a common sequelae
   - E. Pain radiating to the ear is common

3. WHICH OF THE FOLLOWING AGENTS IS USEFUL IN A THERAPEUTIC TRIAL IN PATIENTS WITH FUO?

A. Aspirin
B. Tetracycline
C. Emetine
D. Corticosteroids
E. Chloroquine
F. Isoniazid

ANSWERS

1. (C) This is the description of a patient who had subacute thyroiditis. Until the attending physicians appreciated the significance of the tender thyroid gland, his illness had been felt to represent "FUO" and he was being evaluated for infection, collagen vascular disease and neoplastic disease. Patients with pyogenic thyroiditis are generally much more ill with marked local signs.

2. (A, C, E) Many aspects of subacute thyroiditis suggest a viral etiology although no agent has been isolated. Hashimoto's thyroiditis is felt to represent autoimmune injury to the thyroid gland but subacute thyroiditis is not. A recent report demonstrates the close association of subacute thyroiditis and HLA type-Bw35. The authors speculate that histocompatibility antigen may predispose patients to infectious disease caused by a yet unidentified viral agent in a manner analogous to the predisposition of patients with the HLA B27 antigen to post-Shigella arthritis. Hypothyroidism is not a common sequelae of subacute thyroiditis. Pain radiating to the ear is a frequent complaint of patients with inflammatory diseases of the thyroid gland.

3. (C, E, F) Aspirin and corticosteroids are non-specific anti-inflammatory agents and will modify or even abolish fever due to a number of causes; therefore, they are singularly unattractive for a therapeutic trial. On the other hand, emetine, chloroquine, and isoniazid are quite specific in their activities against _Entamoeba histolytica_, malaria and mycobacteria respectively; therefore, they do recommend themselves to the physician when one of these illnesses is suspected. Tetracycline has broad antimicrobial activity; defervescence in patients with FUO following its use would suggest bacterial infection but not the type or location. It might also interfere with subsequent culture information and is therefore a poor choice.

REFERENCES

1. Hurley JR. Thyroiditis. Disease-a-Month. 1977; 24:5.

2. Nyulassy S, Hnilica P, Buc M, et al. Subacute (deQuervain's) thyroiditis: Association with HLA-Bw35 antigen and abnormalities of the complement system, immunoglobulins and other serum proteins. J Clin Endocrinol Metab 1977; 45:270.

3. Jacoby GA, Swartz MN. Fever of undetermined origin. N Engl J Med 1973; 289:1407.

CASE 23

HISTORY

A 14-year-old black girl is referred with a history of intermittent cough and pulmonary infiltrates. She first consulted her physician 6 months earlier because of fever, malaise and cough of 1 week's duration. A chest roentgenogram at that time revealed a patchy left lower lobe infiltrate, and she was treated with penicillin as an outpatient. All symptoms subsided after 10 days, but she developed low grade fever and cough three months later. Chest roentgenogram at that time revealed a patchy middle lobe infiltrate and right hilar adenopathy. She was again treated with penicillin and her symptoms gradually subsided. Since that time, her only symptom has been rare, intermittent cough. She is referred because her chest roentgenogram remains abnormal.

EXAMINATION

Chest roentgenogram reveals a right hilar mass, felt by the radiologist to represent enlarged hilar nodes and in addition patchy infiltrates in the left upper, and right lower and middle lobes.

LABORATORY DATA

The patient is hospitalized for further evaluation. She remains asymptomatic and afebrile throughout the hospitalization. Hemogram, urinalysis and liver function tests are within normal limits. Multiple examinations of induced sputum for microbiologic and cytologic abnormalities are non-diagnostic. Several skin tests with intermediate strength PPD are negative, and a mumps skin test is positive. Bronchoscopy is normal, but mediastinoscopy reveals enlarged right hilar lymph nodes. Histologic examination of biopsy material from the right hilum shows caseation necrosis but no microorganisms are seen on appropriately stained smears.

QUESTIONS

1. WHICH TWO OF THE FOLLOWING POSSIBILITIES ARE MOST LIKELY AT THIS POINT?
   - A. Adenocarcinoma of the lung
   - B. Asbestosis
   - C. Tuberculosis
   - D. Lymphoma
   - E. Histoplasmosis
   - F. Sarcoidosis

The patient is placed on therapy for tuberculosis. Three weeks after discharge, the results of fungal serology tests, performed on serum obtained while the patient was hospitalized, return. The histoplasmin yeast phase complement fixation antibody titer is positive at a dilution of 1:64, the mycelial phase complement fixing titer is positive as a dilution of 1:32. After 5 weeks' incubation in the appropriate media both sputum and lymphatic tissue obtained from the mediastinum reveal no mycobacterial or fungal growth. Repeated skin tests with PPD have been negative. The patient remains asymptomatic, and her chest roentgenogram is unchanged.

2. APPROPRIATE MANAGEMENT AT THIS POINT IS
   A. continue treatment for tuberculosis
   B. discontinue treatment for tuberculosis; initiate therapy with amphotericin B
   C. continue treatment for tuberculosis and initiate therapy with amphotericin B
   D. discontinue all medications; follow clinically
   E. advise thoracotomy

3. WHICH OF THE FOLLOWING IS/ARE TRUE?
   A. A significant proportion of patients with disseminated histoplasmosis develop adrenal insufficiency
   B. It is very likely that this patient will develop disseminated histoplasmosis at some time during the next 24 months if not treated
   C. Failure of the patient's histoplasmin complement fixation antibody titer to fall to below 1:2 after 8 months would be *a priori* evidence of disseminated disease
   D. Amphotericin B is ineffective against most bacteria because these microorganisms do not have steroids in their plasma membranes
   E. "Selective anergy" to histoplasmin occurs frequently in patient with disseminated histoplasmosis
   F. Sclerosing mediastinitis is a complication of primary infection with *Histoplasma capsulatum*

4. AMPHOTERICIN B IS INDICATED IN WHICH OF THE FOLLOWING DISORDERS?
   A. Most cases of acute pulmonary histoplasmosis
   B. Disseminated histoplasmosis
   C. Chronic cavitary pulmonary histoplasmosis
   D. Whenever *Histoplasma* is isolated from sputum of a patient
   E. Any patient with a positive histoplasmin skin test and calcified granulomata in the spleen

ANSWERS

1. (C, E) The findings of a caseation necrosis of hilar lymph node tissue considerably narrows a previously extensive differential diagnosis.

2. (D) The clinical course, pathology and histoplasmosis serology results point convincingly to the diagnosis of acute primary histoplasmosis. The vast majority of patients with this form of the disease recover within 3 weeks, but the course may be longer as described in the present patient. Treatment with amphotericin B is not indicated for such patients.

3. (A, D, E, F) Adrenal gland involvement is commonly found in patients dying of disseminated histoplasmosis. Clinically significant adrenal insufficiency is less common but should be watched out for in such patients. Patients such as the one described rarely develop disseminated disease, dissemination being more common in children and elderly white males. In the latter group it often occurs years after the primary infection probably at a time when cell-mediated immunity is waning. A histoplasmin complement fixing antibody titer of 1:2 means only that the individual has been infected at some time in the past with _Histoplasma capsulatum_. The mechanism of action of amphotericin B involves binding of the antibiotic with sterol components of plasma membranes. The plasma membranes of fungi and mammalian cells contains sterols, while those of most bacteria do not. Sclerosing mediastinitis is an uncommon but important complication of infection with _H. capsulatum_.

4. (B, C) Acute pulmonary histoplasmosis is a self-limited disease in the vast majority of patients, making Amphotericin B unnecessary. In acute pulmonary histoplasmosis, furthermore, the organism can frequently be recovered from the sputum. The presence of a positive histoplasmin skin test in a patient with calcified granulomata indicates nothing about the activity of the disease.

REFERENCES

1. Polk JW. Treatment of pulmonary histoplasmosis. Dis Chest 1969; 56:149.

2. Brodsky AL, Gregg MB, Lowenstein MS, et al. Outbreak of histoplasmosis associated with the 1970 Earth Day activities. Am J Med 1973; 54:333.

3. Sarosi GA, Voth DW, Dahl BA, et al. Disseminated histoplasmosis: Results of long term follow-up. Ann Intern Med 1971; 75:511.

4. Goodwin RA Jr, Des Prez RM. Histoplasmosis. Am Rev Resp Dis 1978; 117:929.

5. Goodwin RA Jr, Owens FT, Snell JD, et al. Chronic pulmonary histoplasmosis. Medicine (Baltimore) 1976; 55:413.

CASE 24

HISTORY

A 22-year-old male presents because of fever and flank pain. He was in excellent health until one week earlier when he noted low grade fever and mild ache over the right lower postero-lateral rib cage. The pain has become progressively worse every day since that time and he has had chills and fever to 102°F. Epidemiologic history reveals that he works as a transcontinental truck driver, often having occasion to pick up and deliver goods to northern Mexico.

EXAMINATION

Physical examination reveals a moderately ill appearing man with a temperature of 102°F, mild scleral icterus, tender hepatomegaly and point tenderness in the 10th right intercostal space in the posterior axillary line.

LABORATORY DATA

Liver scan reveals a 6 x 6 cm. defect in the posterior portion of the right lobe of the liver.

QUESTIONS

1. WHICH OF THE FOLLOWING STUDIES IS MOST LIKELY TO YIELD INFORMATION WHICH IS SUFFICIENT FOR A PRESUMPTIVE DIAGNOSIS?
   - A. Intravenous cholangiogram
   - B. Liver biopsy
   - C. Ameba hemagglutination inhibition titer
   - D. Carcinoembryonic antigen
   - E. Blood culture
   - F. Hepatic arteriogram
   - G. Alpha-fetoprotein

2. WHICH OF THE FOLLOWING STATEMENTS IS/ARE TRUE?
   - A. Amebic liver abscess most often requires drainage, either surgically or by needle aspiration
   - B. The ameba hemagglutination inhibition titer is usually positive in patients with cecal amebomas
   - C. Pyogenic liver abscess nearly always requires surgical drainage
   - D. *Staphylococcus aureus* is the most common cause of pyogenic liver abscess
   - E. The absence of trophozoites of *Entameba histolytica* from the stool of a patient with liver abscess strongly militates against the diagnosis of amebic liver abscess

ANSWERS

1. (C) The patient most likely has a liver abscess. The absence of a history suggestive of antecedent intra-abdominal illness (such as appendicitis) which would predispose to pyogenic liver abscess and the history of travel into Mexico strongly support the possibility of amebic abscess.

2. (B, C) Many physicians on the African continent, who encounter amebic hepatic abscess with some frequency, routinely aspirate the lesions and have excellent results with combination medical therapy and aspiration. However, most authorities in the United States do not routinely aspirate the lesions and appear to have equally good results with medical therapy alone. The primary indications to aspirate an amebic liver abscess are rupture or signs of impending rupture of the abscess. In contrast, the mortality rate of undrained pyogenic liver abscess approaches 100%; therefore, surgical drainage is mandatory. The ameba hemagglutination inhibition titer, available at the CDC, is an excellent diagnostic test. It is positive in high titer in nearly all cases of invasive amebic disease, including liver abscess and cecal ameboma, but is rarely positive in patients with uncomplicated colonic disease. Pyogenic liver abscess is usually the result of intra-abdominal bacterial disease with spread of infection to the liver via either the portal circulation or the biliary tree. The usual causative microorganisms are intestinal flora. Only about 20% of patients with amebic liver abscess have trophozoites in the stool.

REFERENCES

1. Kragstad DJ, Spencer HC Jr, Healy GR. Amebiasis. New Engl J Med 1978; 298:262.

2. Adams EB, MacLeod IN. Invasive amebiasis. II. Amebic liver abscess and its complications. Medicine 1977; 56:325.

3. Barbour GL, Juniper K Jr. A clinical comparison of amebic and pyogenic abscess of the liver in sixty-six patients. Am J Med 1972; 53:323.

4. DeFord JW. Amebiasis. Newer methods of diagnosis and treatment. South Med J 1973; 66:1149.

5. Sabbaj J, Sutter VL, Finegold SM. Anaerobic pyogenic liver abscess. Ann Intern Med 1972; 77:629.

6. Rubin RH, Swartz MN, Malt R. Hepatic abscess: Changes in clinical, bacteriologic, and therapeutic aspects. Am J Med 1974; 57:601.

CASE 25

HISTORY

A 59-year-old white female was transferred to University Hospital for treatment of tetanus. Ten days previously she lacerated her lower right leg on a stationary "roto-tiller" blade. At a local hospital the wound was cleaned and sutured, and 0.5 ml of tetanus toxoid was administered intramuscularly. Eight days later she noted "stiff jaws" and spasms of her back and abdominal muscles. She was admitted to the local hospital for presumed tetanus and shortly thereafter required emergency tracheostomy because of laryngospasm. She was then transferred to University Hospital for further care.

EXAMINATION

The patient had previously been in good health but had no recollection of primary immunization against tetanus. On admission the vital signs were unremarkable except for temperature of 102°F. Her neck was rigid and she exhibited tetanic spasms of the lower extremities and abdominal musculature. There was a sutured laceration on her right leg without purulent drainage.

Her early hospital course was complicated by profound hemodynamic changes associated with supraventricular tachycardias and marked spontaneous fluctuations in blood pressure.

QUESTIONS

1. WHICH OF THE FOLLOWING STATEMENTS CONCERNING THE ETIOLOGIC AGENT OF TETANUS IS/ARE CORRECT?
   - A. The agent is a gram-positive anaerobic bacillus
   - B. Spore formation occurs and accounts for persistance of the bacteria in soil
   - C. The major virulence factor is a protein exotoxin
   - D. There are 10 distinct antigenic varieties of *Clostridium tetani* but all elaborate an antigenically similar toxin
   - E. The killed whole bacteria is utilized in immunization

2. WHICH OF THE FOLLOWING STATEMENTS ABOUT THE PREVENTION OF TETANUS IS/ARE CORRECT?
   - A. Presently most cases of tetanus arise from serious wounds where there is massive tissue destruction

B. Administration of penicillin G at the time of an injury will reliably prevent tetanus
C. Most cases of tetanus in the United States occur in previously immunized patients
D. A tetanus toxoid booster is sufficient prophylaxis for patients who have received complete immunization within the previous 5 to 10 years
E. Tetanus immune globulin produced in humans carries a small but finite risk of causing hepatitis B

3. WHICH OF THE FOLLOWING STATEMENTS REGARDING THE PATIENT DESCRIBED ABOVE IS/ARE CORRECT?
A. Tetanus immune globulin would have prevented her disease
B. Mortality from tetanus has decreased steadily in the United States and presently stands at around 10%
C. Hypotension and cardiac arrythmias are probably due to autonomic nervous system dysfunction in tetanus
D. Death in tetanus is usually due to a direct effect of the toxin on the myocardium
E. In the United States tetanus is more common in the elderly

ANSWERS

1. (A, B, C, D) Clostridium tetani is a gram-positive anaerobic spore-forming rod; its major toxin, tetanospasmin, is a protein with molecular weight of approximately 145,000. There are 10 distinct antigenic varieties of the bacteria based on flagella antigens but they all elaborate an antigenically similar toxin. Modified toxin, toxoid, is utilized in active immunization. Killed bacteria are not used.

2. (D) Presently most cases of tetanus in the United States occur in patients after relatively minor wounds. Although penicillin G is active against Clostridium tetani, penicillin alone will not prevent tetanus in experimental animals, probably because it does not reach the anaerobic environment where the microorganism multiplies. In the United States today tetanus occurs almost exclusively in patients with incomplete or absent immunization histories. Following full immunization with toxoid, boosters are required only if there has been more than 5 to 10 years since the completion of immunization. Tetanus immune globulin (Homo-Tet®) does not carry hepatitis B agent and is safe although somewhat expensive.

3. (A, C, E) Although a few cases of tetanus have been reported following passive immunization with 250 units of human

tetanus immune globulin, the presently recommended dose of 500 units would almost certainly have prevented tetanus in this patient. Mortality in tetanus has remained around 50% in the United States. The toxin does appear to have an effect on the sympathetic nervous system and this is thought responsible for the severe hemodynamic fluctuations and cardiac arrythmias sometimes noted in patients with this disease. Presently most patients die of infectious complications such as pneumonia. Tetanus in the United States is more common in the elderly because of waning or inadequate immunization.

REFERENCES

1. Weinstein L. In: Prevention of tetanus. Infectious Disease Practice. A Newsletter for the Clinician. 1977; 1:1.

2. Brooks GF, Buchanan TM, Bennett JV. Tetanus toxoid immunization of adults: A continuing need. Ann Int Med 1970; 73:603.

3. Alexander WJ, Cannon NJ, Crow CB, Cobbs CG. Recent experience with tetanus in Alabama. South Med J 1978; 71:1092.

4. Tsueda K, Oliver PB, Richter RW. Medical Intelligence. Cardiovascular manifestations of tetanus. Anesthesiology 1974; 40:588.

CASE 26

HISTORY

A 60-year-old woman is hospitalized because of fever and diarrhea. She was evaluated one month earlier because of congestive heart failure. Findings at that time consisted of blood pressure of 200/125, cardiac enlargement, bilateral basilar rales, and edema of the ankles. She responded quickly to treatment with Digoxin, Lasix and methyldopa. On these medications, she remained asymptomatic, her blood pressure maintained at 160/90 and congestive heart failure completely controlled, until 4 days prior to admission, when she developed chills and fever to 102°F and experienced anorexia and 5 loose, watery stools per day.

EXAMINATION

Physical examination reveals an uncomfortable woman in no acute distress. Her temperature is 100°F, pulse is 80 and regular, blood pressure 160/90 and respiratory rate 14. Funduscopic examination reveals arteriolar narrowing and arterial-venous crossing changes. A grade 2/6 systolic ejection murmur is heard along the left sternal border. The remainder of the physical examination is within normal limits.

LABORATORY DATA

Laboratory examination reveals an hematocrit of 40% and white blood cell count of 8, 000 with 7% eosinophils and an otherwise normal differential. Urinalysis is normal. SGOT is 80, bilirubin 1. 5, and alkaline phosphatase 160. Microscopic examination of the stool reveals no polymorphonuclear leukocytes; the microbial flora consists chiefly of gram-negative bacilli. Intermediate strength PPD elicits 12 millimeters of induration at 48 hours. Electrocardiogram reveals left ventricular hypertrophy; it is unchanged from one month earlier. Chest roentgenogram reveals left ventricular hypertrophy and is also unchanged. Renal function is normal.

QUESTIONS

1. THE MOST LIKELY CAUSE OF THE PATIENT'S ILLNESS IS
   - A. bacterial endocarditis
   - B. reaction to methyldopa
   - C. digitalis intoxication
   - D. disseminated tuberculosis

E. reaction to lasix
F. ascending cholangitis

2. APPROPRIATE INITIAL MANAGEMENT OF THE PATIENT INCLUDES WHICH OF THE FOLLOWING?
A. Withhold digoxin; order serum digoxin level
B. Stop methyldopa
C. Obtain four blood cultures
D. Obtain a sputum culture
E. Evaluate the biliary tree radiographically
F. After blood cultures are obtained, begin ampicillin and gentamicin
G. Begin isoniazid and ethambutol
H. Obtain a stool culture
I. Begin prednisone 60 mg by mouth per day

3. WHICH OF THE FOLLOWING STATEMENTS IS/ARE TRUE?
A. Drug induced fever is not associated with chills
B. Idiosyncratic reactions to methyldopa most often occur during the first few weeks after institution of the drug
C. Procainamide is a common cause of drug-induced systemic lupus erythematosus
D. Eosinophilia is often seen with drug fever due to streptomycin
E. A positive direct and indirect Coombs' test may be seen in patients treated with methyldopa

ANSWERS

1. (B) When we saw this patient, all the choices given were initially considered. The more likely possibilities seemed to be a methyldopa reaction, ascending cholangitis, and perhaps bacterial endocarditis. The combination of fever, diarrhea, mild eosinophilia, and hepatic dysfunction favored a reaction to methyldopa, while the absence of peripheral findings of endocarditis and of right upper quadrant abdominal tenderness made endocarditis and cholangitis, respectively, less likely.

2. (A, B, C, E, H) Since the patient is not currently in heart failure and it is possible that at least some of her symptoms, especially diarrhea, might be due to digitalis intoxication, it seems prudent to withhold digoxin initially. There is a great likelihood, as discussed above, that methyldopa is responsible for all of her current symptoms; it should be discontinued. Since the patient has fever and diarrhea, blood and stool cultures are appropriate; sputum culture is not. In the face of fever and liver dysfunction, we would obtain radiographic

evaluation of the biliary tree. No antimicrobial or anti-inflammatory therapy is indicated.

3. (B, C, D, E) While we are especially suspicious of bacterial infection in patients who present with fever accompanied by chills, virtually any disorder that causes fever may on occasion cause chills. Most drugs which cause a positive Coombs' antiglobulin test (with or without hemolysis) do so by inducing the formation of antibody to the drug; then either the drug binds to the erythrocyte and antibody to the drug, or the drug-antibody complex binds to the erythrocyte. This results in a positive direct Coombs' test but a negative indirect, for only erythrocytes coated with drug and antibody can be agglutinated by anti-immunoglobulin. Methyldopa, on the other hand, induces the production of an antibody which cross-reacts with the Rh_d locus. Therefore, all Rh positive erythrocytes will be agglutinated by anti-immunoglobulin, and both the direct and indirect Coombs' tests will be positive.

REFERENCES

1. Klein HO, Kaminsky N. Methyldopa fever. NY State J Med 1973; 73:448.

2. Cluff LE, Johnson JE III. Drug fever. Prog Allergy 1964; 8:149.

3. Croft JD Jr, Swisher SN Jr, Gilliland BC, et al. Coombs'-test positivity induced by drugs. Mechanisms of immunologic reactions and red cell destruction. Ann Intern Med 1968; 68: 176.

4. Abramson N, Lee DP. Immune hemolytic anemia. Disease-a-Month April, 1974:27-28.

5. Lappat EJ, Cawein MJ. A familial study of procainamide-induced systemic lupus erythematosus. A question of pharmacogenetic polymorphism. Am J Med 1968; 45:846.

CASE 27

HISTORY

A 12-year-old boy was admitted for neurosurgery after a brain tumor had been diagnosed during an outpatient evaluation. One day following surgical exploration of an astrocytoma involving the third ventricular area, the patient became febrile; fever was attributed to the operation. One week later the patient was still febrile and diarrhea was noted. Blood and stool grew Salmonella enteriditis, sub group java. Epidemiologic investigation of the surgical intensive care unit revealed three patients during an eight week period prior to this episode from whom the same salmonella had been recovered, in two patients from blood and stool and in another sputum and urine. The index patient had received no oral food or medication except a tube feeding preparation just prior to onset of diarrhea.

QUESTIONS

1. WHICH MECHANISM(S) IS/ARE PROBABLY RESPONSIBLE FOR THIS OUTBREAK OF SALMONELLA DISEASE IN THE INTENSIVE CARE UNIT?
   A. Contamination of tube feeding or other dietary material by medical personnel who are carriers
   B. Person to person spread by nurses, physicians, etc., not involving dietary material
   C. Contamination of intravenous fluids by the etiologic salmonella
   D. Airborn spread of salmonella, possibly with respirator reservoir contamination

2. WHICH OF THE FOLLOWING IS/ARE TRUE?
   A. Salmonella bacteremia is a common accompaniment of the salmonella gastroenteritis syndrome
   B. Oral ampicillin is appropriate for salmonella gastroenteritis
   C. Most patients with salmonella gastroenteritis will not continue to carry the etiologic microorganism for longer than three months
   D. Antimicrobial resistance in strains of salmonella is commonly mediated by extrachromosomal DNA (plasmids).

3. WHICH OF THE FOLLOWING STATEMENTS ABOUT CLINDAMYCIN COLITIS IS/ARE CORRECT?
   A. This complication occurs in approximately 20% of patients receiving this antibiotic

B. Clindamycin colitis only occurs following oral administration of the drug
C. Clindamycin colitis is due to a direct affect of the antimicrobial agent on the small bowel epithelial cells
D. Clindamycin colitis is due to a toxin elaborated by strains of clostridia
E. Clindamycin colitis responds to therapy with atropine or morphine derivatives

ANSWERS

1. (B) This outbreak at our hospital closely resembles an outbreak reported by Lintz, et al. The pathogenesis was probably person to person spread and did not appear to involve food or medications given by mouth. Most sporadic cases of salmonella gastroenteritis are caused by contamination of food but in the hospital setting, especially in crowded intensive care units, direct person to person spread may occur.

2. (C, D) Bacteremia is actually uncommon in patients with salmonella gastroenteritis. In contrast, bacteremia is common in the salmonella enteric fever syndrome as well as the salmonella bacteremia syndrome. Patients with salmonella gastroenteritis usually do not require antimicrobial therapy. Carriage of salmonella strains following gastroenteritis is unusual after two or three months. Antimicrobial resistance in salmonella is commonly mediated by plasmids.

3. (D) There is disagreement as to the precise incidence of clindamycin colitis but it probably occurs in less than 5% of patients who receive the drug. It has occurred following both oral and parenteral administration. Studies in patients reinforced by data from animal models incriminates toxin elaboration by strains of clostridia and not a direct effect of the antibiotic on the bowel. Clindamycin colitis responds to topical corticosteroids, cholestyramine and oral vancomycin, the latter presumably due to its antibacterial activity against the etiologic clostridia. See the last reference for recent evidence regarding the role of <u>Clostridium difficile</u>.

REFERENCES

1. Lintz D, Kapila R, Pilgrim E, et al. Nosocomial <u>Salmonella</u> epidemic. Arch Int Med 1976; 136:968.

2. Larson HE, Price AB. Pseudomembranous colitis: Presence of clostridial toxin. Lancet 1977; 2:1312.

3. Bartlett JG, Onderdonk AB, Cisneros RL, et al. Clindamycin-associated colitis due to a toxin-producing species of Clostridium in hamsters. J Inf Dis 1977; 136:701.

4. Editorial: Clostridium difficile and chronic bowel disease. Lancet 1980; 1:402.

CASE 28

HISTORY

A 50-year-old man is hospitalized because of pain in the leg associated with purulent drainage. He was in good health until one year earlier when he was hospitalized elsewhere because of pain in the right leg and fever. Roentgenogram of the leg had been normal, and he was treated with penicillin for ten days with defervescence. He did well until three months after discharge from the hospital when he developed pain in the same area and he noted spontaneous discharge of pus. He was treated for a week with penicillin, and the discharge ceased. He again did fairly well until a week prior to the present admission when he developed pain in the leg and low grade fever.

EXAMINATION

Physical examination is normal except for a small sinus tract and tenderness over the area of the tibial plateau. Roentgenogram of the leg shows an area of radiolucency in the tibial plateau consistent with osteomyelitis.

QUESTIONS

1. WHICH TWO OF THE FOLLOWING ORGANISMS ARE MOST LIKELY AS CAUSES OF THIS PATIENT'S ILLNESS?
   A. *Streptococcus pneumoniae*
   B. *Mycobacterium tuberculosis*
   C. *Cryptococcus neoformans*
   D. *Pseudomonas aeruginosa*
   E. *Staphylococcus aureus*

Pus aspirated from the bone grows *Staphylococcus aureus* reported by the laboratory to be intermediately sensitive to penicillin.

2. APPROPRIATE MANAGEMENT WOULD BE
   A. penicillin V 500 mgm PO qid with probenecid
   B. cephalexin 500 mgm PO qid
   C. cloxacillin 500 mgm PO qid
   D. tetracycline 500 mgm PO qid
   E. measure penicillin G MIC or penicillinase production by the organism

3. WHICH OF THE FOLLOWING IS/ARE TRUE?
   A. It is common for radiographic findings to worsen during the first few weeks of appropriate antimicrobial therapy for acute osteomyelitis

B. Spontaneous drainage of pus is a common presenting sign in the initial episode of osteomyelitis
C. Most cases of chronic osteomyelitis can be cured by antimicrobial agents alone provided a high enough dose is given for a sufficient duration
D. Brucellosis may present as vertebral osteomyelitis without an antecedent acute episode of fever and chills
E. In the treatment of penicillin-sensitive Staphylococcus aureus osteomyelitis cultures must be obtained frequently to be certain penicillin resistance has not occurred

4. ANSWER THE FOLLOWING QUESTION BY FILLING IN THE BLANK
The appearance of massive proteinuria in a patient with chronic osteomyelitis should lead one to suspect ____________________.

ANSWERS

1. (B, E) Mycobacterium tuberculosis and Staphylococcus aureus are the most common offenders.

2. (E) Since the organism was reported to be intermediately sensitive to penicillin, it is first necessary to find out if the organism makes penicillinase in order to decide if the drug of choice is penicillin G or a penicillinase-resistant penicillin.

3. (A, D, E) The usual onset is insidious with pain as a major manifestation. A draining sinus is a late manifestation. Chronic osteomyelitis with abscess formation is best treated by a combination of long-term antibiotic therapy and appropriate surgical drainage. Penicillin-sensitive staphylococci do not become penicillin-resistant in clinical situations even with the long term treatment required by osteomyelitis.

4. Amyloidosis.

REFERENCES

1. Waldvogel FA, Medoff G, Swartz MN. Osteomyelitis: A review of clinical features, therapeutic considerations and unusual aspects. New Engl J Med 1970; 282:198, 260, 316.

2. Bell SM. Oral penicillins in the treatment of chronic staphylococcal osteomyelitis. Lancet 1968; 2:295.

3. Koenig MG, Rogers DE. Current status of therapy in acute osteomyelitis. J Am Med Assn 1962; 180:1115.

4. Duma RJ, Kunz LF. Penicillinase production in the evaluation of disc sensitivity testing of staphylococci to penicillin. Am J Clin Path 1970; 53:865.

5. Mollan RAB, Piggot J. Acute osteomyelitis in children. J Bone Joint Surg 1977; 59B:2.

6. Lowe RW, Brooks AL. Hematogenous osteomyelitis. South Med J 1979; 63:1183.

7. West WF, Kelly PJ, Martin WJ. Chronic osteomyelitis. I. Factors affecting the results of treatment in 186 patients. J Am Med Assn 1970; 213:1837.

8. Hedstrom SA. Treatment of chronic staphylococcal osteomyelitis with cloxacillin and dicloxacillin - a comparative study in 12 patients. Scand J Infect Dis 1975; 7:55.

CASE 29

HISTORY

A 65-year-old white man from Chicago is referred because of an abnormal chest roentgenogram. He has been in generally good health, but on questioning admits to slight malaise and a 10 pound weight loss over the previous 6 months.

EXAMINATION

The physical examination is normal.

LABORATORY DATA

Chest roentgenogram reveals bilateral upper lobe infiltrates with small cavities. Sputum smears for acid fast bacilli are negative. Histoplasmosis complement fixation titer is negative. Sputum acid fast culture reveals a mycobacterium which is niacin negative and produces pigment in the light but not in the dark.

QUESTIONS

1. APPROPRIATE ANTIMICROBIAL THERAPY AT THIS POINT IS
   - A. isoniazid, rifampin and ethambutol
   - B. isoniazid and ethambutol
   - C. isoniazid
   - D. isoniazid, rifampin, ethambutol, cycloserine, and ethionamide
   - E. no antimicrobial therapy

2. WHICH OF THE FOLLOWING SKIN TEST RESULTS WOULD BE MOST LIKELY IN THIS PATIENT?
   - A. PPD-S 5 mm; PPD-Y 15 mm; second strength PPD 12 mm
   - B. PPD-S 12 mm; PPD-Y 15 mm; second strength PPD 20 mm
   - C. PPD-S negative; PPD-Y 15 mm; second strength PPD negative
   - D. PPD-S negative; PPD-Y negative; second strength PPD negative
   - E. PPD-S 12 mm; PPD-Y negative; second strength PPD 20 mm

3. WHICH OF THE FOLLOWING STATEMENTS IS/ARE TRUE?

A. Anti-mycobacterial therapy is likely, i. e. has a greater than 80% chance, to cure the patient presented
B. Anti-mycobacterial therapy of disease due to the Battey bacillus is usually curative
C. Scrofula, caused by group II atypical mycobacteria, requires anti-mycobacterial chemotherapy in addition to surgical extirpation of the involved lymph node
D. Swimming pool granuloma, caused by Mycobacterium marinum, usually heals spontaneously without chemotherapy
E. Mycobacterium kansasii causes only pulmonary disease; it does not cause disseminated disease
F. Individuals with atypical mycobacterial pulmonary disease and positive sputum smears should be isolated, just as similar patients with pulmonary disease due to Mycobacterium tuberculosis

ANSWERS

1. (A) The patient has pulmonary disease caused by Mycobacterium kansasii. This mycobacterium is more resistant than is M. tuberculosis to anti-mycobacterial drugs but is not usually resistant in vitro to nearly all agents, as are Mycobacterium avium-intracellulare (Battey bacillus) and the rapid growers. Most patients with pulmonary M. kansasii disease can be cured with medical therapy.

2. (A) PPD-Y would be positive, for it contains antigens of M. kansasii. Many patients who are infected with atypical mycobacteria have small cross-reactions to PPD-S. The most common cause of a negative (<10 mm) intermediate strength (5 TU) PPD and a positive second strength (250 TU) is a cross-reaction with antigens of atypical mycobacteria. Unfortunately, skin test antigens from atypical mycobacteria are not presently available.

3. (A, D) Patients with pulmonary disease due to M. kansasii can usually (85-95%) be cured with antimicrobial therapy, while disease due to the Battey bacillus is much more resistant to treatment. Scrofula does not require chemotherapy. Swimming pool granuloma usually heals spontaneously; however, the rate of healing is increased by treatment with either rifampin or a tetracycline. Atypical mycobacteria generally cause only pulmonary disease but may rarely cause disseminated disease. Atypical mycobacteria are not transmitted from person to person; therefore, patients need not be isolated.

REFERENCES

1. Kubica GP. Differential identification of mycobacteria. Am Rev Resp Dis 1973; 107:9.

2. Runyon EH. Anonymous mycobacteria in pulmonary disease. Med Clin N Am 1959; 43:273.

3. Davidson PT. Treatment and long-term follow-up of patients with atypical mycobacterial infections. Bull Internatl Union Against Tuberc 1976; 51:257.

4. Nicholson DP. Atypical mycobacteria: Features and therapy. Brit J Dis Chest 1976; 70:217.

5. Palmer CE, Edwards LB. Identifying the tuberculous infected. J Am Med Assn 1968; 205:167.

6. Jones PG, Campbell PE. Tuberculous lymphadenitis in childhood: The significance of the anonymous mycobacteria. Brit J Surg 1962; 50:302.

7. Linell F, Norden A. Mycobacterium balnei - A new acid-fast bacillus occurring in swimming pools and capable of producing skin lesions in humans. Acta Tuberc Scand 1954; 33:S1.

8. Izumi AK, Hanke CW, Higaki M. M. marinum infections treated with tetracycline. Arch Dermatol 1977; 113:1067.

CASE 30

HISTORY

A 64-year-old farmer from Alabama was transferred from an outside hospital for evaluation of headache and dizziness of one week duration and lymphocytic meningitis. The patient had a ten year history of rheumatoid arthritis and had been maintained on 15 mg of prednisone daily. Three weeks prior to admission he noted the onset of retroorbital headache followed by dizziness, light-headedness, unsteadiness of gait, nausea and vomiting. On physical examination at the outside hospital he had been lethargic and incoherent. A lumbar puncture there revealed increased white cells, depressed glucose concentration, and budding yeast forms.

QUESTIONS

1. THE MOST LIKELY ETIOLOGIC MICROORGANISM IS
   - A. *Rhizopus oryzae*
   - B. *Nocardia asteriodes*
   - C. *Cryptococcus neoformans*
   - D. *Blastomyces dermatitidis*
   - E. *Coccidioides immitis*

2. WHICH OF THE FOLLOWING DIAGNOSTIC STUDIES SHOULD BE OBTAINED IMMEDIATELY?
   - A. Spinal fluid for cryptococcal antigen
   - B. Spinal fluid culture
   - C. Spinal fluid for routine and fungus complement fixing antibody against coccidioidin
   - D. Serum fungal serologies, e.g. for *Histoplasma capsulatum*, *Blastomyces dermatitidis*, and *Coccidioides immitis*

Cryptococcus neoformans was recovered from the spinal fluid!

3. WHICH OF THE FOLLOWING STATEMENTS REGARDING CRYPTOCOCCAL MENINGITIS IS/ARE CORRECT?
   - A. Cisternal puncture is occasionally useful in diagnosis of cryptocococcal meningitis
   - B. The combination of amphotericin B and 5 flurocytosine is superior to amphotericin B alone for treatment of cryptococcal meningitis
   - C. Amphotericin B dosage should be reduced in patients with renal failure
   - D. 5 flurocytosine is potentially dangerous in patients with impaired renal function

E. The presence of impaired cell mediated immunity predisposes to cryptococcal meningitis, and prejudices the outcome of therapy.

ANSWERS

1. (C) Subacute lymphocytic meningitis with budding yeast forms seen in spinal fluid almost certainly represents cryptococcal disease. Rhizopus oryzae the agent responsible for some forms of mucormycosis only rarely causes primary meningitis. More commonly it presents as rhinocerebral disease in patients with diabetic ketoacidosis or pulmonary infection in severely immunocompromised patients. In addition the agent is a mold and would not be found in the yeast form. Nocardia is a bacteria and would also not appear as a budding yeast. Nocardia may involve the central nervous system; however, the usual site of initial disease is the lung. Blastomyces dermatitidis may cause chronic lymphocytic meningitis but is much less common in this situation than Cryptococcus neoformans. Coccidioides immitis meningitis is an important complication of disease due to that dimorphic fungus. In tissue spherules and not budding yeasts are seen.

2. (A, B, C, D) All of these tests are probably appropriate. Certainly cerebrospinal fluid cryptococcal antigen determination is important in any patient with chronic lymphocytic meningitis. A positive India Ink test would make determination of cryptococcal antigen somewhat superfluous but the antigen titer is still useful in order to quantify response to therapy. One expects the titer of cryptococcal antigen to fall as treatment progresses. In a patient with suspected Coccidioides immitis central nervous system disease the complement fixing antibody against coccidioidin is extremely useful in monitoring response to therapy as well as making the diagnosis since the etiologic yeast is commonly not isolated from cerebrospinal fluid even in advanced central nervous system involvement. Serum antibody levels directed against antigens of Histoplasma capsulatum, Blastomyces dermatitidis and Coccidioides immitis are variably useful. In the case of Coccidioides immitis the presence of serum precipitins reflect early IgM antibody and complement fixing antibodies IgG antibody. The latter are very useful in following patients with Coccidioides immitis disease. Antibodies directed against the yeast and mycelial phase of Histoplasma capsulatum are less helpful but may be useful in suggesting the etiology of an undiagnosed chronic pulmonary infection. It is important to appreciate that many patients with disseminated histoplasmosis have no detectable serum antibody against histoplasmin. Serologies are useless in most instances of serious disease caused by Blastomyces dermatitidis. One exception may be patients with acute symptomatic pulmonary disease.

3. (A, B, D, E) Several studies have demonstrated the usefulness of cisternal puncture in diagnosis of cryptococcal central nervous system disease. The yeast has been found in specimens from the cisterna when it could not be isolated from multiple samples of cerebrospinal fluid from the lumbar area. A controlled multicenter study has demonstrated the efficacy of amphotericin B plus 5 flurocytosine in treatment of cryptococcal meningitis. The use of both drugs allows physicians to reduce the dose of amphotericin B and the duration of therapy; therefore the combination is probably superior to amphotericin B alone. Amphotericin dosage should not be reduced in patients with renal failure since the pharmacology of amphotericin is such that serum levels are not dependent upon renal function. However when patients become severely uremic while receiving amphotericin B, most clinicians tend to reduce the dose or discontinue it for a brief duration of time. It is extremely important to modify dosage of 5 fluorocytosine in patients with renal insufficiency since this agent will accumulate in serum of such patients and severe hematologic disorders such as leukopenia and thrombocytopenia are more common. Nomograms are available for guidance in 5 flurocytosine dosage for patients with renal insufficiency. Approximately one half of patients with cryptococcal meningitis have some disorder of the immune system prior to their disease. Generally impaired cell mediated immunity (disorders of T cell function) seems to predominate in these patients. In addition patients with severe immunologic disturbance such as renal transplant recipients receiving immunosuppressive therapy with corticosteroids and azathioprine respond less favorably to therapy. The report by Morgans et al describes the use of miconazole in this disorder.

REFERENCES

1. Diamond RD. Cryptococcus neoformans. In: Mandell GL, Douglas RG Jr, and Bennett JE, eds. Principles and Practices of Infectious Diseases. New York: John Wiley & Sons, 1979; 2023-34.

2. Diamond RD, Bennett JE. Prognostic factors in cryptococcal meningitis. A study of 111 cases. Ann Intern Med 1974; 80:176.

3. Berger MP, Paz J. Diagnosis of cryptococcal meningitis. J Am Med Assn 1976; 236:2517.

4. Bennett JE, Dismukes WE, Duma RJ, Medoff G, et al. A comparison of amphotericin B alone and combined with flucytosine in the treatment of cryptococcal meningitis. New Engl J Med 1979; 301:126.

5. Morgans ME, Thomas MEM, Mackenzie DWR. Successful treatment of systemic cryptococcosis with miconazole. Brit Med J 1979; 2:100.

6. Anonymous. Treatment of cryptococcosis. Editorial. Lancet 1979; 2:132.

CASE 31

HISTORY

A 21-year-old woman presents because of an illness beginning 10 days previously and characterized by generalized myalgias, headache, chilly sensations and fever. All the symptoms ameliorated 5 days prior to the visit but worsened 2 days later. At that time she also noted fever to 102°F and recurrent chilly sensations. She denies sore throat. Her only medicine has been aspirin for fever. She denies foreign travel.

EXAMINATION

Physical examination reveals an oral temperature of 100°F and mild tenderness in the right upper quadrant. The spleen is not palpable.

LABORATORY DATA

Laboratory work includes a white blood cell count of 5600 with 41% lymphocytes, SGOT of 86 units and a negative mononucleosis spot test, hepatitis B antigen determination and toxoplasma IgM immunofluorescent test.

QUESTIONS

1. WHICH OF THE FOLLOWING DISORDERS ARE MOST LIKELY?
   - A. Infectious mononucleosis
   - B. *Mycoplasma pneumoniae* infection
   - C. Cytomegalovirus infection
   - D. *Toxoplasma gondii* infection
   - E. Malaria

The patient is treated supportively and seen the following week. She is feeling somewhat better, with only low grade afternoon fevers. The white blood cell count is 10,000 with 62% lymphocytes, 3 monocytes, 27 polymorphonuclear leukocytes, 7 band forms and 1 basophil. Her transaminase is 75 units. The complement fixation test for cytomegalovirus infection subsequently rises from less than 1:8 to greater than 1:128 4 weeks after the onset of her illness.

2. WHICH OF THE FOLLOWING STATEMENTS ABOUT CYTOMEGALOVIRUS INFECTION IS/ARE CORRECT?
   - A. Congenital cytomegalovirus infection is associated with a high incidence of serious central nervous system disease
   - B. Congenital cytomegalovirus infection does not occur in infants born to immune mothers

C. Both cytomegalovirus infection and infectious mononucleosis may be associated with the appearance of abnormal serum proteins such as cold agglutinins, rheumatoid factor, and antinuclear antibodies.
D. Cytomegalovirus can be isolated from the urine of most patients with cytomegalovirus mononucleosis syndrome

3. WHICH OF THE FOLLOWING PREDISPOSES PATIENTS TO CYTOMEGALOVIRUS INFECTION?
A. Blood transfusion
B. Leukemia
C. Renal transplantation
D. Bone marrow transplantation

ANSWERS

1. (A, C, D) The atypical pneumonia syndrome is the only human disorder for which the role of Mycoplasma pneumoniae has been clearly established. Malaria would be most unusual in a United States citizen who had no history of foreign travel.

2. (C, D) In contrast to rubella infection during pregnancy, which presents a risk to the fetus only if the mother is not immune, the fetus of the mother with antibodies against cytomegalovirus is not invariably protected from infection. The patient described above had documented cytomegalovirus mononeucleosis syndrome (virus recovered from urine and buffy coat and diagnostic antibody titer rise). This disorder has been described most commonly in females and typically is characterized by fever, liver involvement, and hematologic changes similar to those associated with infectious mononucleosis. Pharyngitis and lymphadenopathy are less common than in infectious mononucleosis and the heterophile test and EB virus antibody studies are negative. Recent investigations suggest that congenital infection with cytomegalovirus is most often not associated with serious central nervous system disease although infection may cause congenital neurological abnormalities.

3. (A, B, C, D) The post-perfusion syndrome of an infectious mononucleosis-like illness which follows cardiopulmonary bypass has been shown to be due to cytomegalovirus infection.

REFERENCES

1. Caul EO. Cytomegalovirus infections after open heart surgery. Lancet 1971; 1:777.

2. Ho M. Cytomegalovirus infections and diseases. Disease-a-Month September, 1978.

3. Nankervis GA, Kumar ML. Diseases produced by cytomegaloviruses. Med Clin NA 1978; 62:1021.

4. Duchowny M, Caplan L, Siber G. Cytomegalovirus infection of the adult nervous system. Ann Neurol 1979; 5:458.

5. Stagno S, Reynolds DW, Huang E-S, et al. Congenital cytomegalovirus infection. New Engl J Med 1977; 296:1254.

6. Jordan MC, Rousseau WE, Stewart JA, et al. Spontaneous cytomegalovirus mononucleosis. Ann Intern Med 1973; 79:153.

7. Weller TH. The cytomegaloviruses: Ubiquitous agents with protein clinical manifestations. New Engl J Med 1971; 285: 203.

8. Klemola E, von Essen R, Wager O, et al. Cytomegalovirus mononucleosis in previously healthy individuals. Five new cases and follow-up of 13 previously published cases. Ann Intern Med 1969; 71:11.

CASE 32

HISTORY

A 16-year-old boy with stage IIB Hodgkin's disease presents because of low grade fever and pain in the left upper quadrant. Six months previously, the diagnosis of Hodgkin's disease had been made by excision biopsy of a left inguinal lymph node. Staging laparotomy revealed involvement of para-aortic nodes, but the liver and the excised spleen were free of disease. He underwent inverted Y irradiation of the para-aortic and inguinal lymphatic chains, was subsequently maintained on cyclic BACOP therapy, and was apparently disease free. He remained asymptomatic until three days prior to admission, when he developed nearly constant left upper quadrant abdominal pain unattended by any other symptoms except low grade fever.

EXAMINATION

Physical examination is normal except for a well healed surgical midline abdominal scar and mild left upper quadrant abdominal tenderness.

LABORATORY DATA

Laboratory evaluation reveals a white blood cell count of 9,000 with a normal differential. The hematocrit and platelet count are normal. Liver function tests and gastrointestinal roentgenograms are normal. On the 2nd hospital day, several vesicular lesions are noted over the left upper quadrant of the abdomen. On the 3rd hospital day, similar lesions appear over the face, trunk, extremities and buccal mucosa, and the patient complains of anorexia and nausea.

QUESTIONS

1. THE MOST LIKELY DIAGNOSIS IS
   - A. cutaneous lymphoma
   - B. disseminated varicella-zoster virus infection
   - C. bacteremia with cutaneous dissemination
   - D. nocardiosis
   - E. disseminated candidiasis
   - F. smallpox
   - G. disseminated <u>Cryptococcus neoformans</u> infection

2. WHICH OF THE FOLLOWING STUDIES IS MOST LIKELY TO BE REWARDING IN MAKING A SPECIFIC DIAGNOSIS?

A. Gram's stain of the vesicular fluid
B. Tzanck preparation of scrapings from the base of a cutaneous lesion
C. Fungus culture of vesicular fluid
D. India ink preparation of the vesicular fluid
E. Serum varicella antibody titer

3. WHICH OF THE FOLLOWING STATEMENTS IS/ARE TRUE?

A. Roughly 15% of healthy adults who contract chicken pox develop varicella pneumonia
B. Varicella pneumonia is micronodular and often resolves with pulmonary calcification
C. People who have had chicken pox may develop herpes zoster (shingles) upon reexposure to a patient with chicken pox
D. On a Tzanck preparation eosinophilic intranuclear inclusions are characteristic of infection with either varicella zoster, herpes simplex 1 or herpes simplex 2 virus
E. Adenine arabinoside appears to be useful in treating cutaneous disseminated herpes zoster infection in immunosuppressed patients
F. Granulomatous carotid arteritis is a rare complication of trigeminal herpes zoster infection
G. The finding of 30 lymphocytes in the cerebrospinal fluid of a patient with trigeminal herpes zoster infection establishes the diagnosis of herpes zoster meningoencephalitis

ANSWERS

1. (B) This is a case of disseminated disease due to varicella-zoster virus, a very serious disease to which patients with disorders of delayed hypersensitivity are unusually susceptible. The clinical picture of localized pain followed by localized and then disseminated vesicular lesions is virtually diagnostic.

2. (B) A Tzanck preparation of scrapings of a lesion is likely to reveal intranuclear inclusions and multinucleated cells diagnostic of infection with a herpes virus. The diagnosis would be quickly confirmed by viral culture.

3. (A, B, C, D, E, F) While radiographically demonstrable involvement of the lung is rare in children with varicella, clinically and radiographically apparent pneumonia occurs in about

1/6 of adults who develop initial infection with varicella. Since localized herpes zoster is a recrudescence of infection in a nerve root, CSF pleocytosis is not unusual and does not necessarily imply involvement of the meninges or brain substance.

REFERENCES

1. Dolin R, Reichman RC, Mazur MH, Whitley RJ. Herpes zoster-varicella infections in immunosuppressed patients. Ann Intern Med 1978; 89:375.

2. Feldman S, Hughes WT, Daniel CB. Varicella in children with cancer: Seventy-seven cases. Pediatrics 1975; 56:388.

3. Triebwasser JH, Harris RE, Bryant RE, et al. Varicella pneumonia in adults: report of seven cases and a review of literature. Medicine 1967; 46:409.

4. Barr RJ, Herten J, Graham JH. Rapid method for Tzanck preparations. J Am Med Assn 1977; 237:1119.

5. Whitley RJ, Ch'ien LT, Dolin R, et al. Adenine arabinoside therapy of herpes zoster in the immunosuppressed. New Engl J Med 1976; 294:1193.

6. Rosenblum WI, Hadfield MG. Granulomatous angiitis of nervous system in cases of herpes zoster and lymphosarcoma. Neurology 1972; 22:348.

CASE 33

HISTORY

This 65-year-old man was referred to University Hospital for a ruptured aortic abdominal aneurysm, acute renal failure and respiratory failure. Several days after admission, at a time when his problems were relatively stable, he began to complain of lower abdominal pain and associated with this was an increased temperature to 103°F. Approximately one week later the abdomen became distended and tympanitic, and because of an abdominal roentgenogram revealing free gas, surgery was performed. At the time of surgery the duodenum was noted to be perforated and there were subphrenic and subhepatic collections of pus.

QUESTIONS

1. WHICH OF THE FOLLOWING PROCEDURES ARE USEFUL FOR DIAGNOSIS OF INTRA-ABDOMINAL ABSCESS?
   - A. Body CT scan
   - B. Gallium scan
   - C. Abdominal roentgenogram (KUB)
   - D. B mode ultrasound
   - E. Barium contrast study

2. WHICH OF THE FOLLOWING ANTIMICROBIAL COMBINATIONS IS REASONABLE THERAPY FOR INTRA-ABDOMINAL ABSCESS, E.G. - PERIAPPENDICAL ABSCESS FOLLOWING PERFORATED APPENDIX?
   - A. Clindamycin and gentamicin
   - B. Penicillin and streptomycin
   - C. Penicillin, chloramphenicol and gentamicin
   - D. Cephalothin and gentamicin
   - E. Erythromycin and metronidazole (Flagyl)

3. WHICH OF THE FOLLOWING STATEMENTS REGARDING SURGICAL DRAINAGE IS/ARE TRUE?
   - A. Placement of drains at the time of intra-abdominal surgery, i.e. cholecystectomy, appendectomy, etc., is clearly associated with a decreased incidence of subsequent wound infection and intra-abdominal abscess
   - B. Pyogenic liver abscess almost always requires drainage
   - C. Within a few days of drain placement only the immediate vicinity of the drain is in continuity with the lumen
   - D. Drains may serve as mechanisms for introduction of resistant microorganisms into the drain site

ANSWERS

1. (A, B, C, D, E) All of these procedures are potentially useful. Gallium 67 is taken up in increased concentrations in areas of acute inflammation; however, because the isotope is secreted into the intestinal tract, accumulations of radioisotope in stool may cause false positive results. Plain roentgenograms of the abdomen as well as barium contrast studies may reveal inflammatory masses or free gas under the diaphram as in this case if hollow viscus perforation has occurred. B mode ultra sound may be helpful in determination of an intra-abdominal mass, however the study is difficult if there is increased bowel gas or distorted anatomy. Recently the total body CT scan has proven very effective for delineation of even small accumulations of inflammatory material and potentially will be very useful in the future.

2. (A, C) 1) Clindamycin together with gentamicin or 2) penicillin, and chloramphenicol with or without gentamicin are the two most common regimens recommended for therapy of intra-abdominal "sepsis" when the disorder has followed intestinal perforation, and the precise microbial etiology is unknown. Both of these combinations offer excellent antimicrobial activity against most anaerobic microorganisms as well as the common aerobic gram-negative bacilli. In addition, penicillin plus gentamicin has good activity against the enterococcus (whose role in the pathogenesis of intra-abdominal abscess is unclear). The combination of cephalothin and gentamicin is relatively ineffective in abscesses caused by or associated with anaerobic bacteria. For that reason it is not an ideal choice early on. Although penicillin and streptomycin was used for years with some success, the emergence of strains of aerobic gram-negative bacilli resistant to streptomicin has resulted in that agent being relatively ineffective at the present time. Erythromycin and metronidazole offer excellent activity against anaerobic microorganisms but are essentially useless for disease caused by aerobic gram-negative bacilli.

3. (B, C, D) There is no convincing evidence that drainage at the time of surgery decreases the incidence of subsequent intra-abdominal abscess since within a short time only the area immediate to the drain is in continuity with the exterior. Drains may even serve to introduce resistant microorganisms. Liver abscess caused by pyogenic bacteria almost always requires surgical drainage. In contrast amebic liver abscess may be managed without drainage.

REFERENCES

1. Levison ME. Peritonitis and intra-abdominal abscess. In: Mandell GL, Douglas RG Jr, and Bennett JE, eds. Principles and Practice of Infectious Diseases. New York: John Wiley & Sons, 1979, 609-43.

2. Altemeier WA, Culbertson WR, Fullen WD, et al. Intra-abdominal abscesses. Am J Surg 1973; 70:125.

3. Bartlett JG, Louie TJ, Onderdonk AB, et al. Whither the enterococcus? 15th ICAAC, September 24-26, 1975 Washington, DC, Abstract #297.

4. Finegold SM. Abdominal and perineal infections. In: Anaerobic Bacteria in Human Disease. New York: Academic Press, 1977; 257.

5. Ralph ED, Kirby WMM. Unique bacterial action of metronidazole against _Bacteriodes fragilis_ and _Clostridium perfringens_. Antimicrob Ag Chemother 1975; 8:409.

6. Haller JA Jr, Shaker IJ, Donahoo JS, et al. Peritoneal drainage versus non-drainage for generalized peritonitis from ruptured appendicitis in children: A prospective study. Ann Surg 1973; 177:595.

7. Cerise EJ, Pierce WA, Diamond DL. Abdominal drains: Their role as a source of infection following splenectomy. Ann Surg 1970; 171:764.

8. Thadepalli H, Gorbach SL, Broido PW, et al. Abdominal trauma, anaerobes, and antibiotics. Surg Gynec Obstet 1973; 137:270.

9. Ozeran RS. Subdiaphragmatic abscess: Diagnosis and treatment. Am Sur 1967; 33:64.

10. Roberts EAB, Nealon TF Jr. Subphrenic abscess: Comparison between operative and antibiotic management. Ann Surg 1974; 180:209.

11. Katzman DO. Combined liver-lung gamma imaging in subphrenic abscess. S Afr Med J 1976; 50:1367.

12. Caffee HH, Watts G, Mena I. Gallium 67 citrate scanning in the diagnosis of intra-abdominal abscess. Am J Surg 1977; 133:665.

13. Hill BA, Yamaguchi K, Flynn JJ, et al. Diagnostic sonography in general surgery. Arch Surg 1975; 110:1089.

14. Blair DC, Carroll M, Silva J, Fekety R Jr. Localization of infectious processes with gallium citrate Ga 67. J Am Med Assn 1974; 230:82.

15. Halasz NA. Subphrenic abscess: Myths and facts. J Am Med Assn 1970; 214:724.

16. Lorber B. Bacteriology of intra-abdominal infection. Surg Clinics of N. A. 1975; 55:1349.

17. Daffner RH, Halber, MD, Morgan, CL, et al. Computed tomography in the diagnosis of intra-abdominal abseceses. Ann Surg 1979; 189:29.

18. Anonymous. Peritoneal drainage. Lancet 1979; 2:941.

CASE 34

HISTORY

A 45-year-old man sustained a shotgun wound to the right calf. Initial therapy consisted of cleaning the wound, excision of necrotic skin and muscle, and administration of tetanus toxoid. The next day, he has low grade fever and complains of severe pain in the leg. Twelve hours thereafter, crepitus is noted over the gastrocnemius and roentgenograms of the leg reveal gas in muscle planes. Gram's stain of exudate from the wound reveals a large gram-positive bacilli.

QUESTIONS

1. THE MOST IMPORTANT THERAPEUTIC MODALITY IS
   A. Transferring the patient immediately to a center equipped with a hyperbaric oxygen chamber
   B. Administration of high dose penicillin G
   C. Administration of polyvalent gas gangrene antitoxin
   D. Wide excision of all devitalized tissue
   E. Administration of tetanus antitoxin

2. THE DISTINCTION BETWEEN CLOSTRIDIAL CELLULITIS AND CLOSTRIDIAL MYONECROSIS IS BEST MADE BY
   A. palpation of the involved part
   B. x-ray of the involved part
   C. exploration of the wound with direct visualization of fascia and muscle
   D. blood culture
   E. the initial response to treatment with penicillin

3. WHICH OF THE FOLLOWING STATEMENTS IS/ARE TRUE?
   A. Necrotizing fasciitis with gas formation is nearly always due to clostridia
   B. Progressive synergistic bacterial gangrene is necrotizing cellulitis due to *Staphylococcus aureus* and anaerobic streptococci and often begins at the site of abdominal retention sutures
   C. The isolation of *Clostridium perfringens* from a wound demands wide debridement and administration of penicillin
   D. Clostridia may occasionally enter the blood stream via an inapparent site in the gastrointestinal tract

4. MATCH THE FOLLOWING MICROORGANISMS WITH THE MECHANISM OF ACTION OF THEIR RESPECTIVE TOXINS:

1. *Clostridium perfringens*
2. *Clostridium tetani*
3. *Clostridium botulinum*
4. Enteropathogenic *Escherichia coli*
5. *Corynebacterium diphtheriae*

A. Blocks elongation factor II.
B. Inhibits internuncial activity
C. Presynaptic blockade
D. Lecithinase
E. Elevates cyclic AMP levels within cells

ANSWERS

1. (D) Clostridia, being strict anaerobes, require an anoxic environment in order to grow. Once they gain a foothold in a devitalized area, both toxins released by the bacterium and the inflammatory response itself help to create anoxic conditions in adjacent tissues, so the organisms can invade them as well. Spread from a small area to involvement of an entire limb and the trunk may occur with remarkable rapidity, so it is mandatory to halt the process by excising all devitalized tissue.

In centers equipped with hyperbaric chambers, remarkable improvement in ischemic areas has resulted from hyperbaric oxygen therapy, and this is a therapeutic modality which deserves consideration. However, in patients with fairly localized disease, such as the patient described, hyperbaric oxygen therapy should not be employed to the exclusion of surgical debridement. Unless a hyperbaric chamber were almost immediately available, we would recommend operating on the patient first and considering the advisability of hyperbaric oxygen later. The patient should receive penicillin and, depending upon his immunization status, tetanus prophylaxis as well; but these are of secondary importance. Gas gangrene antitoxin is not indicated.

2. (C) Clostridia may simply colonize a wound without causing disease, may cause cellulitis, may cause myonecrosis, and may even cause bacteremia. Clostridia can be cultured from about 30% of traumatic wounds. The vast majority of these are simply colonized and no ill effects result. Gas in the tissues implies that clostridia (or other anaerobes) have gained a foothold and are causing disease but does not distinguish between cellulitis, a fairly benign disorder requiring only antimicrobial therapy and incision and drainage, and myonecrosis, a serious disorder requiring excision of involved tissues. This distinction

can be made with confidence only by direct visualization of tissue at operation.

3. (B, D) A variety of bacteria, chiefly anaerobes, but often in conjunction with aerobes, are capable of causing gas forming soft tissue infections. Clostridia are present in low titer in the normal colon. Patients with necrotic intestinal lesions, usually carcinoma, occasionally develop spontaneous clostridial bactermia.

4. (A) 5
(B) 2
(C) 3
(D) 1
(E) 4

REFERENCES

1. Altemeier WA, Fuller WD. Prevention and treatment of gas gangrene. J Am Med Assn 1971; 217:806.

2. Fowler DL, Evans LL, Mallow JE. Monoplace hyperbaric therapy for gas gangrene. J Am Med Assn 1977; 238:882.

3. Slack WK, Hanson CG, Chew HER. Hyperbaric oxygen in the treatment of gas gangrene and clostridial infection. Brit J Surg 1969; 56:505.

4. Gorbach SL, Thadepalli H. Isolation of clostridium in human infections: Evaluation of 114 cases. J Infect Dis 1975; 131: 581.

5. Finegold SM, Bartlett JG, Chew AW, et al. Management of anaerobic infections. Ann Intern Med 1975; 83:375.

6. Alpern RJ, Dowell VR Jr. Clostridium septicum infections and malignancy. J Am Med Assn 1969; 209:385.

CASE 35

HISTORY

A 23-year-old white female was transferred to the medical service because of fever and bacteremia. She had been admitted to the neurosurgery service one week previously with a seizure disorder, and an A-V malformation of the parietal lobe had been discovered. Two days prior to transfer erythema and tenderness had appeared at the site of an indwelling intravenous catheter and fever was noted. Two blood cultures obtained prior to transfer grew Staphylococcus aureus.

EXAMINATION

Physical examination on transfer revealed a toxic, febrile woman with nuchal rigidity, conjunctival and palatal petechiae, bilateral inspiratory rales, a harsh blowing apical systolic murmur, and mild confusion. The intravenous catheter was still in place and, in addition to signs of local inflammation, a purulent exudate was present. There was no history of hypersensitivity to penicillin.

QUESTIONS

1. INITIAL MANAGEMENT SHOULD INCLUDE WHICH OF THE FOLLOWING?
   - A. Removal of the polyethylene catheter with Gram stain of exudate and culture of the catheter tip
   - B. Exploratory proximal phlebotomy
   - C. High dose aqueous penicillin G
   - D. Parenteral penicillinase resistant semi-synthetic penicillin, e.g. methicillin or nafcillin
   - E. Lumbar puncture
   - F. Additional blood cultures

On the next day blood cultures obtained at the time of transfer also grew Staphylococcus aureus and spinal fluid examination revealed pleocytosis, depressed glucose concentration, and Gram-positive cocci in clumps.

2. WHICH OF THE FOLLOWING STATEMENTS IS/ARE TRUE REGARDING THE APPROPRIATE MANAGEMENT OF PATIENTS WITH STAPHYLOCOCCAL BACTEREMIA?
   - A. Patients whose bacteremia emanates from an identifiable intravascular site may not require therapy for as long as other patients with staphylococcal bacteremia

B. In the United States less than 20% of strains of S. aureus are presently susceptible to penicillin G
C. Approximately 20% of strains of S. aureus are presently resistant to semi-synthetic penicillins such as methicillin and nafcillin
D. Newer cephalosporins such as cefazolin may not be as active in vitro against large inocula of S. aureus as semi-synthetic penicillins such as nafcillin

3. WHICH OF THE FOLLOWING STATEMENTS ABOUT STAPHYLOCOCCAL CENTRAL NERVOUS SYSTEM INFECTION IS/ARE TRUE?
A. Staphylococcal meningitis usually results from antecedent staphylococcal bacteremia
B. Subdural empyema is commonly caused by S. aureus
C. A variety of antistaphylococcal antimicrobial agents including clindamycin and cephalothin are satisfactory for treatment of staphylococcal central nervous system disease
D. Mycotic aneurysms of the intracranial vessels do not appear to be as common in staphylococcal endocarditis as in endocarditis caused by viridans streptococci

ANSWERS

1. (A, B, D, E, F) This case describes a patient who developed staphylococcal bacteremia, endocarditis and meningitis because of an infected intravenous catheter. Initial therapy should include removal of the catheter with Gram stain and cultures. We believe that additional blood cultures are especially useful immediately after removal of an intravascular foreign body prior to the initiation of antimicrobial therapy in order to document whether or not bacteremia persists after the foreign body is out of the circulation. Surgical debridement of infected IV catheter sites is not always required, but when there is obvious proximal suppuration, it is necessary. A penicillinase resistant penicillin must be employed initially for therapy of suspected or proven staphylococcal disease, since the vast majority of strains are presently resistant to penicillin G. A lumbar puncture is appropriate in this situation to determine if meningitis is present.

2. (A, B, D) Iannini and Crossley reported that staphylococcal bacteremia associated with a removable focus may not require as long a course of antimicrobial therapy as staphylococcal bacteremia occurring in the absence of an identifiable site of local disease. Watanakunakorn and Baird have rebutted this argument by presenting data showing the rather frequent

complication of staphylococcal endocarditis as a result of staphylococcal catheter infection. We believe the results of blood cultures obtained just after removal of an infected intravenous catheter as well as physical examination directed especially toward identification of sites of metastatic localization should influence the total duration of antistaphylococcal therapy. Only rarely are strains of Staphylococcus aureus presently isolated in the United States found to be resistant to semi-synthetic, penicillinase resistant penicillins such as nafcillin. Cephalosporins, especially cefazolin, do appear to be more susceptible to an inoculum effect.

3. (A, B, D) Staphylococcal meningitis may result from extension of staphylococcal disease from sinuses or paracranial sites into the subarachnoid space or from bacteremia as in this instance. The latter is probably more common. Staphylococcal sinusitis, especially involving the frontal sinus, is the most common antecedent event preceding subdural empyema. Clindamycin and cephalothin are not appropriate antimicrobial agents for therapy of staphylococcal meningitis since neither predictably results in adequate central nervous system levels. Mycotic aneurysm seems to be a more common complication of streptococcal endocarditis than staphylococcal endocarditis, possibly because of a longer duration of illness prior to diagnosis in the former disease.

REFERENCES

1. Iannini PB, Crossley K. Therapy of Staphylococcus aureus bacteremia associated with a removable focus of infection. Ann Int Med 1976; 84:558.

2. Watanakunakorn C, Baird IM. Staphylococcus aureus bacteremia and endocarditis associated with a removable infected intravenous device. Am J Med 1977; 63:253.

3. Stein JM, Pruitt BA Jr. Suppurative thrombophlebitis. A lethal iatrogenic disease. N Engl J Med 1970; 282:1452.

CASE 36

HISTORY

A 25-year-old man presents because of fever and headache of 12 hours' duration. Past medical history reveals that he has had three episodes of meningitis in the past two years. These episodes were managed at another hospital and records are not immediately available. According to the patient, he was treated with an antibiotic intravenously for each episode and was asymptomatic within three to four days of initiation of therapy. He does not know whether or not a microorganism was cultured from the cerebrospinal fluid. Between episodes he has been totally well. There is no prior history of head trauma.

EXAMINATION

Physical examination reveals an acutely ill appearing man with a temperature of 103°F and marked nuchal rigidity. The remainder of the physical examination, including detailed neurologic examination, is normal.

LABORATORY DATA

Lumbar puncture reveals an opening pressure of 160; 2000 white cells, 85% of which are polymorphonuclear; glucose of 52; and protein of 90. Gram's stain, acid fast smear, and India ink preparation of the cerebrospinal fluid do not reveal any microbial forms. Roentgenograms of the skull, mastoids, sinuses, and chest are normal.

QUESTIONS

1. YOU WOULD
   - A. hospitalize the patient and observe, planning to repeat the lumbar puncture in 12-24 hours
   - B. send the patient home with instructions to return if the symptoms worsen
   - C. begin therapy with 20,000,000 units per day of aqueous penicillin intravenously
   - D. begin therapy with 12 gm/day of ampicillin intravenously
   - E. begin therapy with 4-6 gm/day of chloramphenicol intravenously
   - F. begin therapy with isoniazid and rifampin in appropriate doses
   - G. begin therapy with nafcillin 12 gm/day intravenously

The next day the patient feels generally better; the following information is available: Cerebrospinal fluid and blood cultures are sterile. On each of the three prior hospitalizations, the cerebrospinal fluid formula was similar to that of the admission specimen and no microorganism was isolated. The patient was treated with penicillin on each occasion and was well in three to four days. No specific diagnosis was made.

On reviewing the cerebrospinal fluid Gram's stain you note that in addition to numerous polymorphonuclear leukocytes there are occasional "epithelioid" cells.

2. THE PATIENT'S ILLNESS IS MOST LIKELY
   A. carcinomatous meningitis
   B. lymphomatous meningitis
   C. Behcet's disease
   D. Mollaret's disease
   E. recurrent bacterial meningitis, probably as a result of an occult basilar skull fracture

3. WHICH OF THE FOLLOWING IS/ARE TRUE?
   A. The absence of a history of significant head trauma rules out basilar skull fracture with a mucosal-meningeal communication as a cause of recurrent bacterial meningitis
   B. A glucose determination on nasal secretions is useful in detecting cerebrospinal fluid rhinorrhea
   C. About 10% of patients with brain abscess have cerebrospinal fluid formulas suggestive of pyogenic meningitis
   D. The clinical course of patients with recurrent pneumococcal meningitis caused by a meningeal communication with the skin or with the nasal mucosa is often more benign than that of other patients with pneumococcal meningitis
   E. The natural history of Mollaret's meningitis is characterized by increasingly frequent episodes of meningitis

ANSWERS

1. (C, E) There are several unusual features of the patient's illness. First, he has had several prior episodes of what seem to be bacterial meningitis. This raises the possibility that he may have an anatomic defect permitting recurrent entry of bacteria into the subarachnoid space. An example of such defects is an inapparent basilar skull fracture with a dural tear and communication between the meninges and the nasopharynx; another example is a congenital tract between the skin and the subarachnoid space. Second, the CSF glucose is not depressed and the protein not as elevated as one would expect with bacterial meningitis. And third, no bacteria are seen on Gram's stain. With pneumococcal meningitis resulting in an inflammatory response of 2000 white blood cells/mm^3, it would be most unusual not to find pneumococci on a Gram's stained smear of CSF.

Nevertheless, while it is far from clear what the cause of the patient's illness is, the likelihood of bacterial infection of the central nervous system is sufficiently great that he should be treated immediately.

2. (D) The history of recurrent, sterile meningitis characterized by infiltration of the meninges with several thousand neutrophils/mm^3, the brief courses of illness, and especially the finding of epithelial cells in the CSF establish the diagnosis of Mollaret's disease, a rare disorder of unknown course.

3. (B, C, D) While most patients who have basilar skull fractures and mucosal-meningeal communications have a history of major head trauma, there are patients described who have developed this complication after only minimal injuries. The presence of glucose in nasal secretions suggests a CSF leak. The characteristic CSF formula in patients with brain abscess is a few hundred cells, a mixture of neutrophils and lymphocytes; normal glucose; and protein of about 150 mg%. However, in about 10% of patients, the CSF formula more closely resembles that of bacterial meningitis. In our experience, these are patients whose abscesses are immediately adjacent to a ventricle. For reasons that are not clear, recurrent pneumococcal meningitis appears to be a less severe disease in patients who have meningeal-pharyngeal communications than in patients who develop pneumococcal meningitis for other reasons. The natural history of Mollaret's meningitis is characterized by increasingly infrequent episodes of meningitis.

REFERENCES

1. Hermans PE, Goldstein NP, Wellman WE. Mollaret's meningitis and differential diagnosis of recurrent meningitis. Report of a case, with review of the literature. Am J Med 1972; 52: 128.

2. Haynes BF, Wright R, McCracken JP. Mollaret meningitis. A report of three cases: J Am Med Assn 1976; 236:1967.

3. Galloway WH, Chambers W. Pneumococcal meningitis: skull defects as aetiological factor. Lancet 1953; 2:68.

4. Hand WL, Sanford JP. Posttraumatic bacterial meningitis. Ann Intern Med 1970; 72:869.

CASE 37

HISTORY

A 67-year-old man is brought to the emergency room because of confusion. The patient has a long history of recurrent sinusitis. Five days prior to presentation he complained of headache and malaise and had low grade fever. These symptoms persisted, and the day before presentation his family noted intermittent confusion. He has received no medicine during the previous month.

EXAMINATION

Physical examination reveals a stuporous, disoriented man with slight nuchal rigidity. His temperature is 102°F and pulse rate 110; respirations and blood pressure are normal. Funduscopic examination and the remainder of the general physical examination are normal. Neurologic examination reveals a slight drift of the left arm, slight weakness of the left arm and leg, left homonymous hemianopsia, and a left Babinski sign.

QUESTIONS

1. THE MOST IMPORTANT INITIAL MANEUVER IS
   - A. lumbar puncture
   - B. roentgenograms of the sinuses
   - C. CAT scan of the brain
   - D. initiation of therapy with nafcillin and chloramphenicol
   - E. right carotid arteriogram

CAT scan with contrast reveals a low density right fronto-temporal lesion surrounded by a ring of high density.

2. THE MOST LIKELY DIAGNOSIS IS
   - A. herpes simplex encephalitis
   - B. infected brain tumor
   - C. non-infected brain tumor
   - D. brain abscess
   - E. encephalitis caused by a virus other than herpes simplex

3. WHICH OF THE FOLLOWING STATEMENTS IS/ARE TRUE?
   - A. Anaerobic bacteria play a role in most brain abscesses
   - B. Clindamycin is an excellent choice for treatment of brain abscess
   - C. Prompt drainage of infected paranasal sinuses is an important adjunctive procedure in the management of a patient who has sinusitis and central nervous system infection

D. Culture of cerebrospinal fluid from patients with brain abscess usually reveals anaerobic streptococci
E. The advent of CAT scan has reduced by about 80% the need for cerebral arteriography and has virtually eliminated the need for pneumoencephalography

ANSWERS

1. (D) The patient presents with signs of a central nervous system infection and focal neurologic signs. The risk of cerebellar tonsillar herniation from lumbar puncture is too high in our judgement to perform a lumbar puncture immediately without further definition of intra-cranial dynamics. While it is true that one wishes to obtain appropriate material for culture before initiating antimicrobial therapy, he does so only if there is no or minimal risk. Furthermore, it is most unlikely that the patient presented has bacterial meningitis; brain abscess and herpes encephalitis are much more likely. In these disorders, one will not obtain diagnostic information from examination of CSF. In the case of the patient presented, we would be sufficiently concerned about the adverse consequences of delaying antimicrobial therapy for even an hour so that we would first initiate therapy then immediately obtain a CAT scan. We would perform lumbar puncture only if the CAT scan indicated it were safe to do so.

2. (D) While tumors cannot be distinguished from brain abscesses by CAT scan, the combination of the clinical presentation and CAT scan findings makes brain abscess by far the most likely diagnosis. The CAT scan in herpes simplex encephalitis usually reveals a low density temporal lesion; however, the lesion is not surrounded by high density.

3. (A, C, E) Anaerobic bacteria are present in 80-85% of brain abscesses. While clindamycin is an excellent antimicrobial agent for most infections caused by anaerobes, it does not cross the blood-brain barrier sufficiently well ever to be used for treatment of CNS infections. It is important not only to treat CNS infection but also to drain the source of the infection, such as paranasal sinuses. In brain abscess, bacteria are usually localized to the brain substance and do not gain access to the CSF; therefore, cultures of CSF are almost invariably sterile.

REFERENCES

1. Samson DS, Clark K. A current review of brain abscess. Am J Med 1973; 54:201.

2. Brewer NS, MacCarthy CS, Wellman WE. Brain abscess: a review of recent experience. Ann Intern Med 1975; 82:571.

3. Weisberg LA. Computed tomography in the diagnosis of intracranial disease. Ann Intern Med 1979; 91:87.

CASE 38

HISTORY

A 7-month-old Italian boy with cyanotic congenital heart disease had repair of an endocardial cushion defect 3 days ago. You are consulted because of a blood culture which is said to show gram-positive cocci in the clusters.

EXAMINATION

On examination the baby is lethargic and has a temperature of 104°F. The sternotomy wound is erythematous and has a small area of fluctuance at its cephalad end. The heart examination has not changed since surgery. A chest x-ray film shows the mediastinum to have widened appreciably in the last 48 hours.

QUESTIONS

1. IMMEDIATE MANAGEMENT WOULD INDICATE
   A. aspiration of the wound at the area of fluctuance
   B. re-exploration
   C. institution of antibiotics
   D. blood cultures
   E. lumbar puncture

2. THE GRAM STAIN OF THE ASPIRATED PUS ALSO SHOWS GRAM-POSITIVE COCCI. THE APPROPRIATE ANTIBIOTIC WOULD BE
   A. erythromycin
   B. penicillin G
   C. a penicillinase-resistant penicillin
   D. gentamicin
   E. a cephalosporin

You start the baby on methicillin. The next day the bacteriology laboratory calls to say that the organism in the baby's blood and wound aspirate is *Staphylococcus aureus* but is resistant to methicillin. The baby undergoes drainage of a wound abscess and anterior mediastinitis.

3. YOU WOULD SWITCH THE BABY FROM METHICILLIN TO
   A. a cephalosporin
   B. a tetracycline
   C. chloramphenicol
   D. vancomycin
   E. clindamycin

4. WHICH OF THE FOLLOWING IS/ARE TYPES OF PENICILLIN-RESISTANCE FOUND IN STAPHYLOCOCCI?

A. Drug inactivation by a β-lactamase
B. Intrinsic resistance without drug inactivation
C. Tolerance, when the MBC of penicillin is many times higher than the MIC

ANSWERS

1. (A, B, C, D) The widened mediastinum indicates the wound infection has spread to deeper tissues producing mediastinitis.

2. (C) Staphylococcus aureus must be assumed to be penicillin-resistant until proven otherwise. A cephalosporin may be used if the child is allergic to penicillins.

3. (D) Methicillin-resistant Staphylococcus aureus are almost always resistant to cephalosporins, tetracyclines, and chloramphenicol. A few are also resistant to clindamycin. All are sensitive to vancomycin. We used vancomycin and added rifampin to raise the serum bactericidal activity to titers of 1:16.

4. (A, B, C) β-lactamase hydrolysis of penicillin is the most common form of resistance, occurring in the majority of isolated strains. Methicillin resistance is a form of intrinsic resistance, found much more commonly in Europe than in the U. S.

REFERENCES

1. Hoeprich PD, Benner EJ, Kayser FH. Susceptibility of methicillin-resistant Staphylococcus aureus to twelve antimicrobial agents. Antimicrob Agents Chemother 1969;104.

2. Cook FV and Farran E, Jr. Vancomycin revisited. Ann Intern Med 1978; 88:813.

3. Kayser FH. Methicillin-resistant staphylococci: 1965-75. Lancet 1975; 2:650.

4. Esposito AL and Gleckman RA. Vancomycin: A second look. J Am Med Assn 1977; 238:1756.

5. Culliford AT, et al. Sternal and costochondral infections following open heart surgery. A review of 2,594 cases. J Thorac Cardiovasc Surg 1976; 72:714.

6. Denny AE, Peterson LR, Gerding DN, Hall WH. Serious staphylococcal infections with strains tolerant to bactericidal antibiotics. Arch Intern Med 1979; 139:1026.

CASE 39

HISTORY

A 47-year-old male abattoir worker is hospitalized because of fever. He was in excellent health until a week earlier when he noted malaise and fever to 101°F. The next day these symptoms were worse and he developed generalized headache. All symptoms progressively worsened and his temperature has been 104°F continuously for the past 48 hours.

EXAMINATION

Physical examination reveals an acutely ill man with a temperature of 104°F and pulse rate of 84. The spleen tip is palpable. The remainder of the physical examination is normal.

LABORATORY DATA

The white cell blood count is 4500 with 40% lymphocytes and 60% neutrophils. Blood cultures obtained at the time of admission reveal a gram-negative bacillus.

QUESTIONS

1. THE MOST LIKELY CAUSATIVE MICROORGANISM IS
   A. *Shigella sonnei*
   B. *Salmonella java*
   C. *Escherichia coli*
   D. *Pseudomonas aeruginosa*
   E. *Bacteroides fragilis*
   F. *Brucella abortus*

Stool and urine cultures reveal the same microorganism as grew in blood cultures. Appropriate antimicrobial therapy is administered and the patient improves. Six weeks after cessation of antimicrobial therapy the same microorganism is cultured from the patient's stool. The patient is asymptomatic and the physical examination normal.

2. APPROPRIATE MANAGEMENT OF THE PATIENT AT THIS POINT INCLUDES
   A. ampicillin
   B. chloramphenicol
   C. oral cholecystogram
   D. barium examination of the colon
   E. none of the above

3. WHICH OF THE FOLLOWING STATEMENTS IS/ARE TRUE?

A. Salmonella typhi is most often acquired by man from another human
B. Other salmonellae are most often acquired by man from another human
C. Salmonella gastroenteritis generally requires antimicrobial therapy
D. Shigella gastroenteritis generally requires antimicrobial therapy
E. Typhoid fever is generally a biphasic illness
F. Trimethoprim-sulfamethoxazole is a useful antimicrobial regimen for treatment of typhoid fever caused by strains resistant to chloramphenicol and ampicillin
G. Amoxicillin is an appropriate substitute for ampicillin in the treatment of shigellosis

ANSWERS

1. (B) Abattoir workers are heavily exposed to salmonellae, brucellae and other bacteria. The clinical features of this patient's illness - consisting of sustained high fever, relative bradycardia, and splenomegaly - are strongly suggestive of enteric fever due to salmonella. While brucellosis is a possibility, the height of his fever and the fact that fever is sustained are against that diagnosis.

2. (E) It is not uncommon for patients who have salmonella infections to excrete the organism in the stool for several weeks after recovery from illness; they require no treatment. Patients who continue to excrete salmonellae for many months usually harbor the organism in the gallbladder; these patients should be evaluated for gallbladder disease. If gallstones are found, then consideration should be given to treating the patient with a prolonged course of ampicillin and removing the gallbladder.

3. (A, D, F, G) Antimicrobial therapy is indicated for patients with salmonella gastroenteritis only when bacteremia is documented or suspected. The vast majority of patients with salmonella gastroenteritis recover spontaneously after a few days; antimicrobial therapy may actually prolong the carrier state in such patients. Most authorities agree that patients with shigellosis should receive antimicrobial therapy. Despite the fact that amoxicillin has a microbial spectrum nearly identical to that of ampicillin, amoxicillin is not effective against shigellae.

REFERENCES

1. Saphia I, Winter JW. Clinical manifestations of salmonellosis in man: An evaluation of 7779 human infections identified at the New York Salmonella Center. New Engl J Med 1957; 256: 1128.

2. Cherubin CE, Neu HC, Imperato PJ, et al. Septicemia with non-typhoid salmonella. Medicine 1974; 53:365.

3. Freitag JL. Treatment of chronic typhoid carriers by cholecystectomy. Public Health Rep 1964; 79:567.

4. Phillips WE. Treatment of chronic typhoid carriers with ampicillin. J Am Med Assn 1971; 217:913.

5. Chin TDY. Therapy of salmonellosis. Ration Drug Ther 1976; 10:1.

6. Aserkoff B, Bennett JV. Effect of antibiotic therapy in acute salmonellosis on the fecal excretion of salmonellae. New Engl J Med 1969; 281:636.

7. Gilman RH, Terminel M, Levine MM, et al. Comparison of trimethoprim-sulfamethoxazole and amoxicillin in therapy of chloramphenicol-resistant and chloramphenicol-sensitive typhoid fever. J Infect Dis 1975; 132:630.

8. Nelson JD, Haltalin KC. Amoxicillin less effective than ampicillin against Shigella in vitro and in vivo: Relationship of efficacy to activity in serum. J Infect Dis 1974; 129:S222.

CASE 40

HISTORY

A 44-year-old white man was admitted to the hospital because of hoarseness and dysphasia. These symptoms had first appeared approximately eight months prior to admission and after two months of illness he was seen by an ear, nose and throat physician who found and biopsied a laryngeal mass. Microscopic examination of the resected tissue revealed budding yeasts with inflammatory tissue "compatible with histoplasmosis". The patient was lost to followup and then readmitted for repeat diagnostic studies.

EXAMINATION

On physical examination the patient's vital signs were normal and he was hoarse. Otherwise the examination was unremarkable as was the admitting laboratory work. On the second hospital day the patient was taken to the operating room where direct laryngoscopy was performed, along with biopsy of the laryngeal mass. Again the pathologic report revealed budding yeast, this time said to be consistent with blastomycosis.

QUESTIONS

1. WHICH OF THE FOLLOWING ARE CLINICAL INDICATIONS FOR INITIATION OF THERAPY FOR BLASTOMYCOSIS?
   - A. Visualization of the characteristic budding yeast forms in a biopsy of a skin lesion
   - B. Culture of _Blastomyces dermatitidis_ from sputum in a patient with a pulmonary infiltrate
   - C. A positive skin test and elevated serologic titers in a patient with a pulmonary infiltrate consistent with blastomycosis
   - D. Budding yeast forms consistent with blastomycosis from a prostate biopsy which shows granulomatus inflammation

2. ANSWER THE FOLLOWING TRUE OR FALSE
   - A. Blastomycosis tends to be more severe in patients with suppression of T cell function
   - B. Hydroxystilbamadine still has an important role in the therapy of blastomycosis
   - C. Outbreaks of blastomycosis among dogs may herald the onset of disease in humans
   - D. Blastomycosis can be easily recovered from soil especially if samples are obtained near pigeon or starling roosts

3. WHICH OF THE FOLLOWING STATEMENTS REGARDING ACUTE PULMONARY BLASTOMYCOSIS IS/ARE TRUE?

A. This entity has been described in several outbreaks and resembles acute pulmonary histoplasmosis
B. Therapy is unnecessary
C. Serologic studies have proven useful in the diagnosis of acute pulmonary blastomycosis
D. Person to person spread has been common

ANSWERS

1. (A, B, D) Presently most investigators believe that blastomycosis involving the skin is a result of dissemination presumably from a pulmonary site. Patients with this disorder require systemic amphotericin B therapy. Rarely a sporotrichoid variety of blastomycosis has been observed in patients following skin inoculation, for example following a laboratory accident, but this is distinctly uncommon. Most patients with cutaneous blastomycosis have disseminated infection. The presence of a chest roentgenogram consistent with blastomycosis and a positive sputum culture is sufficient evidence to require initiation of amphotericin therapy. Blastomyces dermatitidis is not a saphrophyte and when isolated from sputum represents invasive disease in the respiratory tract in most instances. On the other hand the presence of a positive skin test and elevated serologic titers are not sufficiently sensitive or specific to justify initiation of amphotericin therapy in a patient with an abnormal chest roentgenogram. Treatment should only be initiated when the microorganism has either been seen or grown from sputum or observed in a biopsied specimen from the lung. Most physicians would feel justified in treating patients with granulomatous prostatitis and a biopsy reveals budding yeasts consistent with blastomycosis.

2. (A, C) Most all deep fungal diseases tend to be more aggressive in patients with disorders of cell mediated immunity (T cell disorders), and blastomycosis is no exception. Hydroxystilbamadine, which was the first effective chemotherapeutic agent for blastomycosis, has just about been replaced by amphotericin B. Hydroxystilbamadine may have a role in patients who relapse following amphotericin B therapy. There have been reports of epidemics of blastomycosis among dogs which have preceded disease among humans in the same geographic area. Blastomyces dermatitidis has only rarely been recovered from soil. Its ecologic niche is unclear, although there is a suggestive occupational hazard among those who work in earth moving and timber operations, especially in the southeastern United States.

3. (A, B) An atypical pneumonia syndrome caused by Blastomyces dermatitidis has been well described in a couple of instances. It resembles acute pulmonary histoplasmosis. Therapy is unnecessary, and most patients have been diagnosed in retrospect. In contrast to patients with disseminated blastomycosis, patients with acute pulmonary disease have positive blastomycin skin tests and positive serologies. Serologic studies and skin tests for blastomycosis are singularly worthless in patients with disseminated disease. As is the case with most deep fungal infections, person to person spread does not occur.

REFERENCES

1. Fields BT Jr. Blastomyces dermatitidis. In: Mandell GL, Douglas RG JR, and Bennett JE, eds. Principles and Practices of Infectious Diseases. New York: John Wiley & Sons, 1979; 2047-53.

2. Sarosi GA, Hammerman KJ, Tosh FE, Kronenberg RS. Clinical features of acute pulmonary blastomycosis. New Engl J Med 1974; 290:540.

3. Landay ME, Schwarz J. Primary cutaneous blastomycosis. Arch Dermatol 1971; 104:408.

4. Sarosi GA, Eckman MR, Davies SF, Laskey WK. Canine blastomycosis as a harbinger of human disease. Ann Int Med 1979; 91:733.

5. Sarosi GA, Davies SF. Blastomycosis. Am Rev Resp Dis 1979; 120:911.

CASE 41

HISTORY

A 34-year-old accountant presents to the emergency room because of headache and fever of three days' duration. Three days previously he first noted the onset of a severe generalized headache, which has become progressively worse since. Shortly thereafter he began to feel feverish. The day prior to admission his wife noted mild confusion and irritability.

EXAMINATION

On physical examination the blood pressure is 110/70, pulse rate 120, respiratory rate 24, and temperature 103°F. The general physical examination is otherwise unremarkable. Neurologic examination reveals disorientation to time and place, combativeness, generalized hyperreflexia and bilateral Babinski signs.

LABORATORY DATA

Lumbar puncture reveals an opening pressure of 300 mm, 200 cells (90% lymphocytes, 10% polymorphonuclear leukocytes), sugar of 85 mg%, (con-comitant blood sugar of 110 mg%) and protein of 65 mg%. Gram's stain, acid fast stain, and India ink preparations were negative.

QUESTIONS

1. THE COURSE, PHYSICAL EXAMINATION AND CSF ARE MOST CONSISTENT WITH A DIAGNOSIS OF
   - A. bacterial meningitis
   - B. tuberculosis meningitis
   - C. viral encephalitis
   - D. multiple sclerosis
   - E. cryptococcal meningitis

The patient's condition deteriorates and by the third hospital day he is comatose. There are no lateralizing signs, but an EEG shows bitemporal slow waves in addition to a generalized abnormality. A brain CT scan showed cerebral edema, most marked in the left fronto-temporal area.

2. WHICH OF THE FOLLOWING IS/ARE TRUE?
   - A. Brain abscess is not a consideration, for the cerebrospinal fluid sugar was normal and cultures remain sterile

B. Brain biopsy and culture may well reveal a specific viral etiology which is treatable
C. One should begin systemic amphotericin B therapy, for cryptococcal meningitis is likely
D. Serial complement fixation antibody titers to adenovirus will probably show a marked rise
E. Serum anti-herpesvirus antibody titers will be a useful diagnostic test

3. WHICH OF THE FOLLOWING STATEMENTS CONCERNING ENCEPHALITIS IS/ARE TRUE?
A. Full recovery from mumps encephalitis is common
B. Full recovery from herpes simplex encephalitis is common
C. Both idoxuridine and cytosine arabinoside have been shown to be effective in the treatment of mumps encephalitis
D. Adenine-arabinoside (vidarabine, Ara-A) is an effective form of treatment for herpes simplex encephalitis
E. Side effects of vidarabine are frequent and include stomatitis, alopecia, and leukopenia

ANSWERS

1. (C) The sudden onset of encephalitis together with the cerebrospinal fluid findings is most suggestive of a viral etiology, although cryptococcal meningitis may rarely present with such a short duration of symptoms. Untreated bacterial or tuberculous meningitis is extremely unlikely because of the normal cerebrospinal fluid sugar. In fact, the patient had herpes simplex encephalitis.

2. (B) In a patient like this, brain abscess must always be considered even in the absence of lateralizing signs since the history and cerebrospinal fluid findings are compatable with that diagnosis. Spinal fluid cultures are usually sterile in patients with brain abscess unless the abscess communicates with the ventricular system. Brain biopsy with pathologic examination and culture is the diagnostic method of choice for detecting herpes simplex encephalitis. With rare exceptions a physician should not begin treatment for disseminated fungal disease or fungal meningitis unless the organism has been seen or cultured. Because of the tendency of herpesvirus to cause latent infection with periodic reactivation, positive serum antibody titers are insufficient to diagnose herpes virus encephalitis.

3. (A, D) Unfortunately the mortality of herpes simplex encephalitis is quite high, and permanent neurologic sequelae are

common among survivors. Both idoxuridine and cytosine arabinoside are ineffective in the treatment of herpes simplex encephalitis. There is no effective agent for mumps encephalitis. Vidarabine has little toxicity itself. The large fluid volumes required to administer it, however, may worsen cerebral edema.

REFERENCES

1. Whitley RJ, Soong S-J, Dobin R, et al. Adenine arabinoside therapy of biopsy-proved herpes simplex encephalitis. New Engl J Med 1977; 297:289.

2. Nahmias AJ, Roizman B. Infection with herpes-simplex viruses 1 and 2. New Engl J Med 1973; 289:667, 719, 781.

3. Miller JR, Horter DH. Acute viral encephalitis. Med Clin N A 1972; 56:1393.

4. Levine DP, Lanter CB, Lerner AM. Simultaneous serum and CSF antibodies in herpes simplex virus encephalitis. J Am Med Assn 1978; 240:356.

5. Williams BB, Lerner AM. Some previously unrecognized features of herpes simplex virus encephalitis. Neurology 1978; 28:1193.

CASE 42

HISTORY

A 26-year-old black man presents because of fever and cough. He received a cardaveric renal transplant six months previously and had been doing well on prednisone and cyclophosphamide until one week previously when he developed fever to 102°F and non-productive cough. Since that time, he has had daily fever of 102°F and worsening cough, productive of moderate quantities of yellow sputum.

EXAMINATION

Physical examination reveals a moderately ill appearing man with a temperature of 102°F. Rales and signs of consolidation are present over the right lower lobe.

LABORATORY DATA

Chest roentgenogram reveals a pneumonic infiltrate with a small cavity in the lateral basal segment of the right lower lobe. Gram's stain of the sputum reveals small gram-positive cocci in branching filamentous chains. Acid fast smear of the sputum reveals these forms to be weakly acid fast.

QUESTIONS

1. THE MOST LIKELY DIAGNOSIS IS
   - A. streptococcal pneumonia
   - B. staphylococcal pneumonia
   - C. Mycobacterium tuberculosis
   - D. atypical mycobacterial disease
   - E. nocardia pneumonia
   - F. actinomycosis
   - G. aspergillus pneumonia

The patient is begun on appropriate therapy. Three days later, he is generally better but his hematocrit has fallen from 36 to 24%. Further evaluation reveals that the serum haptoglobin is 0.

2. WHICH OF THE FOLLOWING STUDIES IS/ARE LIKELY TO BE ABNORMAL?
   - A. Sugar water test for paroxysmal nocturnal hemoglobinuria
   - B. Erythrocyte glucose-6-phosphate dehydrogenase level
   - C. Direct Coombs' test
   - D. Indirect Coombs' test
   - E. Hemoglobin electrophoresis
   - F. Antinuclear antibodies
   - G. None of the above

3. WHICH OF THE FOLLOWING ANTIMICROBIAL AGENTS SHOULD A PATIENT WITH GLUCOSE-6-PHOSPHATE DEHYDROGENASE DEFICIENCY AVOID?

A. Chloroquine
B. Primaquine
C. Chloramphenicol
D. Nitrofurantoins
E. Nalidixic acid
F. PAS
G. Sulfonamides

4. MATCH THE FOLLOWING BACTERIA AND FUNGI WITH THE APPROPRIATE DESCRIPTIVE PHRASE. USE EACH CHOICE ONLY ONCE.

1. Cryptococcus neoformans
2. Coccidioides immitis
3. Nocardia asteroides
4. Actinomyces israeli
5. Histoplasma capsulatum
6. Blastomyces dermatitidis
7. Aspergillus species
8. Phycomycetes (Mucor)

A. Cause of allergic pulmonary disease
B. Sudden onset of central nervous system symptoms and signs
C. Determination of a microbial antigen in the cerebrospinal fluid is helpful in diagnosis
D. Determination of antibody to the organism in the cerebrospinal fluid is helpful in diagnosis
E. Anaerobic
F. Yeast may be seen in wet preparation of sputum from patients with pneumonia caused by this organism
G. Ulcer of larynx in an elderly white male farmer
H. Causes extensive pulmonary thrombosis when associated with invasive pulmonary disease

ANSWERS

1. (E) The findings on Gram's stain and acid fast smear of the sputum are classical for Nocardia asteroides. Actinomyces israeli is indistinguishable from nocardia on Gram's stain but is less likely to be acid fast. The clinical setting, i.e. a patient

with depressed delayed hypersensitivity; the clinical and radiographic findings; and the sputum findings establish the diagnosis of nocardia pulmonary infection.

2. (G) The most likely cause of hemolytic anemia in this patient is that he has underlying erythrocyte G-6-PD deficiency and that sulfadiazine triggered hemolysis. Nevertheless, if erythrocyte G-6-PD is assayed at a time when 1/3 of his erythrocytes have been lysed, the value obtained is likely to be normal, for most of his G-6-PD deficient cells have been lysed and those that remain are likely to be normal.

3. (B, C, D, E, G)

4. (A) 7
(B) 3
(C) 2
(D) 1
(E) 4
(F) 6
(G) 5
(H) 8

All of the fungi that cause disseminated disease can cause laryngeal ulceration, but <u>Histoplasma capsulatum</u> is much more likely to do so than the rest, our Case 40 notwithstanding. Invasive disease caused by both aspergillus and phycomyces is associated with pulmonary thrombosis. Mucor should be selected over aspergillus only because there is another choice for aspergillus.

REFERENCES

1. Young LS, Armstrong D, Blevins A, Lieberman P. Nocardia asteroides infection complicating neoplastic disease. Am J Med 1971; 50:356.

2. Maderazo EG, Quintiliani R. Treatment of nocardial infection with trimethoprim and sulfamethoxazole. Am J Med 1974; 57:671.

3. Kucers A. The use of antibiotics. Philadelphia: JB Lippincott Co., 1972; 322-323.

4. Golbert TM, Patterson R. Pulmonary allergic aspergillosis. Ann Intern Med 1970; 72:395.

5. Bennett JE, Dismukes WE, Duma RJ, et al. A comparison of amphotericin B alone and combined with flucytosine in the treatment of cryptococcal meningitis. New Engl J Med 1979; 301:126.

6. Pappagianis D. Coccidioidomycosis. In: Samter M. Immunological Diseases, Second Edition. Boston: Little, Brown and Co., 1975.

7. Smith JW, Utz JP. Progressive disseminated histoplasmosis. A prospective study of 26 patients. Ann Intern Med 1972; 76:557.

8. Young RC, Bennett JE, Vogel CL, et al. Aspergillosis. The spectrum of the disease in 98 patients. Medicine 1970; 49:147.

CASE 43

HISTORY

A ten-year-old Mexican child is brought to the emergency room because of fever and sore throat of six days' duration.

EXAMINATION

Examination reveals a temperature of 101°F. There is a dirty gray membrane over both tonsils and the posterior pharynx.

QUESTIONS

1. IN CONDUCTING THE REMAINDER OF THE PHYSICAL AND LABORATORY EVALUATION, YOU WOULD FOCUS YOUR ATTENTION MOST CLOSELY ON WHICH FOUR OF THE FOLLOWING ORGANS OR AREAS?
   - A. The central nervous system
   - B. The cranial nerves
   - C. Peripheral nerves
   - D. Liver
   - E. Kidneys
   - F. Lungs
   - G. The airway
   - H. Joints
   - I. Heart
   - J. Skeletal muscles
   - K. Gastrointestinal tract
   - L. Skin
   - M. Genitalia

Further history reveals that the child had one "baby shot" at 6 months of age but no subsequent immunizations. The remainder of the physical examination is normal and initial laboratory data are normal except for a white blood cell count of 11,000 with a slight left shift.

2. AFTER OBTAINING THROAT CULTURES AND INCOCULATING THE SAMPLE ON A LOEFFLER'S SLANT AND BLOOD AGAR PLATE, YOU WOULD
   - A. treat the patient symptomatically and ask the parents to call the next day regarding the results of the culture
   - B. treat the patient with benzathine penicillin and ask him to return for follow-up in 3 days
   - C. hospitalize the patient and begin treatment with penicillin
   - D. hospitalize the patient and begin treatment with erythromycin
   - E. hospitalize the patient and begin treatment with diphtheria antitoxin and erythromycin

3. WHICH OF THE FOLLOWING STATEMENTS IS/ARE TRUE?

A. Carriers of Corynebacterium diphtheriae should be treated for 10-12 days with either penicillin or erythromycin
B. A positive Schick test indicates immunity to diphtheria toxin
C. Blood cultures are commonly positive in diphtheria
D. The quantity of toxin elaborated is dependent upon both the extent and location of the diphtheritic membrane
E. The highest mortality in diphtheria occurs in patients with laryngeal involvement
F. Evidence of intoxication with diphtheria toxin may occur in patients with Corynebacterium diphtheriae skin infection
G. Toxin elaboration by Corynebacterium diphtheriae is dependent upon the presence of a bacteriophage in the bacterium

ANSWERS

1. (B, C, G, I) The chief concern is that the patient may have diphtheria, the most serious consequences of which are airway obstruction, myocarditis, and peripheral neuropathy including cranial neuropathy.

2. (E) The likelihood of diphtheria is sufficiently great that the patient should be treated immediately. The most important therapeutic modality is not antimicrobial therapy but administration of antitoxin, though we would administer erythromycin as well.

3. (A, D, E, F, G) Carriers should be treated as indicated with erythromycin. The Schick test is performed by injecting a small amount of toxin (0.1 ml) intradermally; a positive reaction indicates susceptibility, or lack of immunity, to the toxin. Bacteremia is very rare in diphtheria and when present is usually due to secondary invaders such as group A streptococci. Laryngeal diphtheria carries the highest mortality rate, even in patients treated with antitoxin. Diphtheria skin lesions have been observed in troops in the tropics. They appear as ulcers with a leathery black eschar that may give rise to myocardial and neurologic sequelae in the same manner as pharyngeal diphtheria. Corynebacterium diphtheriae which are not lysogenized with the appropriate phage do not produce toxin.

REFERENCES

1. Dobie RA, Tobey DN. Clinical features of diphtheria in the respiratory tract. J Am Med Assn 1979; 242:2197.

2. McCloskey RV, Eller JJ, Green M, et al. The 1970 epidemic of diphtheria in San Antonio. Ann Intern Med 1971; 75: 495.

3. McCloskey RV, Green M, Eller J, Smilack J. Treatment of diphtheria carriers: Benzathine penicillin, erythromycin, and clindamycin. Ann Intern Med 1974; 81:788.

4. Liebow AA, MacLean PD, Bumstead JH, Welt LG. Tropical ulcers and cutaneous diphtheria. Arch Intern Med 1946; 78:255.

5. Freeman VJ. Studies on the virulence of bacteriophage-infected strains of Corynebacterium diphtheriae. J Bact 1951; 61:675.

CASE 44

HISTORY

A 15-year-old girl was admitted because of weakness of the lower extremities. Five days previously, while sitting in the yard and stretching her legs, she notices a "pop" in the posterior mid-thoracic area and subsequently developed a dull aching pain at that site which radiated anteriorly bilaterally. Four days later, she began to notice a tingling sensation in both lower extremities. During the next 24 hours, numbness and tingling gradually spread upward to the mid-thoracic level and she experienced weakness in both lower extremities.

EXAMINATION

On physical examination, the patient was an obese, white female with profound weakness of both lower extremities. Temperature was 102°F and respirations were primarily diaphragmatic at 18/min. There was mild nuchal rigidity and pain on anterior flexion of the neck. There was point tenderness over the spine at the T5 level. The remainder of the general physical examination was unremarkable. Neurologic examination revealed flaccid paralysis of the lower extremities with absent tendon reflexes. She was anaesthetic below the level of T5.

LABORATORY DATA

The WBC was 13,000 with a normal differential. Otherwise, admission laboratory work was unremarkable.

QUESTIONS

1. WHICH OF THE FOLLOWING DISORDERS SHOULD BE INCLUDED IN THE INITIAL DIAGNOSIS?
   - A. Brain abscess
   - B. Herpes virus encephalitis
   - C. Spinal epidural abscess
   - D. Guillian-Barre syndrome
   - E. Acute multiple sclerosis

A LP revealed a spinal block and a myelogram delineated a lesion at T8.

2. THERAPY AT THIS TIME SHOULD INCLUDE WHICH OF THE FOLLOWING?
   - A. Antiviral therapy directed against herpes virus
   - B. Broad spectrum antimicrobial agents

C. Immediate neurosurgical exploration of the dorsal spine at the involved site
D. Brain scan
E. Blood cultures

Thoracic laminectomy revealed an epidural abscess. Gram stain of abscess material showed numerous polymorphonuclear leukocytes and gram-positive cocci in clumps.

3. WHICH OF THE FOLLOWING STATEMENTS CONCERNING SPINAL EPIDURAL ABSCESS IS CORRECT?
A. This patient's course, which evolved over 5 days, is unusual for this condition
B. The thoracic spine is the most common site of spinal epidural abscess
C. Gram-negative enteric bacilli are presently the most common etiologic bacteria responsible for this disorder
D. Spinal epidural abscess consititues a neurosurgical emergency. Diagnosis and drainage should be carried out immediately
E. Point tenderness at the involved site is actually uncommon

ANSWERS

1. (C) Spinal epidural abscess is the only likely diagnosis. Brain abscess usually causes upper motor neuron signs and would not be associated with a sensory level. Herpes virus encephalitis causes fever, disordered consciousness, and occasionally seizures and/or focal signs suggesting a mass lesion in the temporal lobe. Guillian-Barre syndrome causes ascending paralysis but sensory nerves are not involved. Acute multiple sclerosis, which may be similar to acute allergic encephalomyelitis in animals, can produce central and peripheral nervous system signs and symptoms. However, one would not expect point tenderness over the spine.

2. (C, E) Antiviral therapy directed against herpes would be inappropriate. One could probably justify initiation of antimicrobial therapy, especially an agent directed against staphylococci, e.g. nafcillin. On the other hand, if surgery were planned immediately, physicians could await results of Gram stain. Blood cultures are appropriate since staphylococcal spinal epidural abscess is frequently a result of bacteremia. A brain scan would be unnecessary.

3. (B, D) This patient's course is actually quite typical of spinal epidural abscess. The thoracic spine is the most common

site of the process and Staphylococcus aureus is the most common etiologic bacterium. This disorder represents a neurosurgical emergency. Point tenderness at the involved site is common. The combination of spinal root pain, point tenderness and neurologic findings in the lower extremities should strongly suggest this diagnosis.

REFERENCES

1. Baker AS, Ojemann RG, Swartz MN, et al. Spinal epidural abscess. N Engl J Med 1975; 293:463.

2. Schlossberg D, Schulman JA. Spinal epidural abscess. South Med J 1977; 70:669.

CASE 45

HISTORY

A 56-year-old black woman was admitted to the hospital in diabetic ketoacidosis. Her diabetes was promptly controlled with insulin. A fever to 101°F began on the third hospital day and has continued for 6 additional days. Except for the fever, she is asymptomatic.

EXAMINATION

Physical examination reveals her temperature to be 101.2°F with a pulse rate of 100. Conjunctival vessels are injected. The optic fundi are normal. A soft systolic ejection murmur is heard along the left sternal border.

LABORATORY DATA

Laboratory data include a WBC count of 8300 with 43% neutrophils and 17% bands. The alkaline phosphatase is elevated slightly to 140 IU/L, but the SGOT and bilirubin are normal. Whereas a chest film on admission was normal, it now shows widespread finely nodular infiltrates.

QUESTIONS

1. OF THE TESTS BELOW, WHICH IS THE MOST USEFUL IN CONFIRMING THE DIAGNOSTIC IMPRESSION?
   A. Sputum cytology
   B. Blood cultures
   C. Serologic tests for Legionnaires' disease
   D. PPD skin test
   E. Heterophile antibody titer

An ophthalmologist called to evaluate her conjunctivitis notes not only injected conjunctival blood vessels but also flare and cells in the anterior chamber with keratic precipitates, consistent with an iritis. Her PPD skin test produces 25 mm induration at 48 hours. Her fever has continued without symptoms. A bone marrow biopsy shows no granulomata.

2. YOU WOULD NOW
   A. start systemic steroid treatment for the iritis
   B. perform a liver biopsy
   C. begin INH and rifampin
   D. perform an open lung biopsy
   E. start broad-spectrum antibiotics

On the 4th day of anti-tuberculous treatment she defervesces and remains afebrile for the next week.

3. THE APPROPRIATE MANAGEMENT NOW SHOULD BE
   A. open lung biopsy
   B. liver biopsy
   C. repeat bone marrow biopsy
   D. continue anti-tuberculous treatment
   E. begin systemic corticosteroid treatment

4. RIFAMPIN MAY PRODUCE WHICH OF THE FOLLOWING?
   A. Rapid emergence of resistance if the drug is used alone
   B. Hepatitis
   C. Thrombocytopenia
   D. Light-chain proteinuria
   E. Deafness

ANSWERS

1. (D) The pattern of diffuse, finely nodular infiltrates represents the miliary pattern characteristic of disseminated tuberculosis. Its appearance over a matter of days excludes malignancy as the cause.

2. (C) Topical steroids are used for the granulomatous iritis.

3. (D) Empiric anti-tuberculous treatment of patients with FUO was frequently used as a diagnostic procedure. This patient's prompt and persistent defervescence in the face of her clinical presentation satisfactorily made the diagnosis of miliary tuberculosis, so that no further efforts at diagnosis are required.

4. (A, B, C, D)

REFERENCES

1. Berger HW, Samortin TG. Miliary tuberculosis: Diagnostic methods with emphasis on the chest roentgenogram. Chest 1970; 58:586.

2. Cucin RL, Coleman M, Eckardt JJ, Silver RT. The diagnosis of miliary tuberculosis: Utility of peripheral blood abnormalities, bone marrow and liver needle biopsy. J Chron Dis 1973; 26:355.

3. Gelb AF, Leffler C, Brewin A, et al. Miliary tuberculosis. Am Rev Respir Dis 1973; 108:1327.

4. Graber CD, Patrick CC, Galphin RL. Light chain proteinuria and cellular mediated immunity in rifampin treated patients with tuberculosis. Chest 1975; 67:408.

5. Grieco MH, Chmel H. Acute disseminated tuberculosis as a diagnostic problem. Am Rev Resp Dis 1974; 109:554.

6. Munt PW. Miliary tuberculosis in the chemotherapy era, with a clinical review in 69 American adults. Medicine 1971; 51:139.

7. Sahn SA, Neff TA. Miliary tuberculosis. Am J Med 1974; 56:495.

8. Sanders WE. Rifampin. Ann Intern Med 1976; 85:82.

CASE 46

HISTORY

This 49-year-old man was admitted to a local hospital because of fever and myalgias. One week previously, while watching television, he noted the sudden onset of chills and muscle aches, mainly involving the large muscle group of the back and legs. During the next several days he thought he had fever and noted continued muscle aches. One day prior to admission he measured his temperature, found it was 103°F, and sought medical assistance.

The patient worked as a drapery cleaner. In addition he had recently removed the floor of the bathroom of a house into which he had moved. He denied exposure to ticks or rodents.

EXAMINATION

On physical examination the patient was febrile with a temperature of 104°F orally. Otherwise there were no other remarkable findings. The patient remained in the hospital for three days during which time his fever spiked to 103-104°F daily. On the third day he signed out against medical advice, but returned to the hospital four days later because of the persistance of the fever, nausea and malaise. On this second admission the physical exam revealed a temperature of 104°F but no focal signs.

LABORATORY DATA

Laboratory evaluation demonstrated a white blood cell count of 6000 with 69% polymorphonuclear leukocytes, 9% bands, 14% lymphocytes, and 8% monocytes. The platelet count was 140, 000. The SGOT was 575, I. U. and alkaline phosphatase 215 I. U. Hepatitis B antigen was not present in serum and the monospot test and toxoplasma IgM IFA were negative.

QUESTIONS

1. WHICH OF THE FOLLOWING DISORDERS IS MOST <u>UNLIKELY</u> IN THIS PATIENT?
    - A. Legionnaires' disease
    - B. Cytomegalovirus mononucleosis syndrome
    - C. EB virus infection, i.e. infectious mononucleosis
    - D. Rickettsial disease
    - E. Leptospirosis

Four days after the second hospitalization the patient developed a macular erathematous rash mainly involving the trunk. This persisted for two or three days and then faded. Febrile agglutinins revealed the OX-19 titer was 1:20 and the OX-K was 1:80.

2. WHICH OF THE FOLLOWING STATEMENTS IS/ARE TRUE?

A. An OX-19 titer of greater than 1:80 on a single serum specimen is diagnostic of rickettsial disease
B. A "saddle back" fever curve is frequently observed in patients with lymphocytic choriomeningitis, leptospirosis and dengue
C. Leptospira organisms may be grown from urine of patients with Weils disease if appropriate media is utilized
D. Sulfonamide therapy may increase the severity of rickettsial illness
E. Q fever is not associated with a rise in the Weil-Felix titer

Repeat febrile agglutinins obtained two weeks later revealed the OX-19 titer was 1:1280 and the complement fixation test for antibody to R. typhi (formerly R. mooseri) revealed a titer rise from 0 on the first specimen to 1:256 on the second, confirming the diagnosis of murine typhus.

3. WHICH OF THE FOLLOWING STATEMENTS ABOUT MURINE TYPHUS IS/ARE CORRECT?

A. The rash of murine typhus is usually less prominent than the rash of Rocky Mountain spotted fever, is generally truncal and may last only a day or two, or in fact may be absent in as many as 40% of the patients with the disease
B. The vector for murine typhus is the rat flea
C. In the United States murine typhus is reported almost exclusively from the far West
D. Liver function abnormalities, as noted in this patient, are distinctly unusual in patients with murine typhus

ANSWERS

1. (A) While Legionnaires' disease may begin with non-specific signs and symptoms including nausea, vomiting and fever, pneumonia is present in most all seriously ill patients. Cytomegalovirus, EB virus and Toxoplasma gondii may all cause a mononucleosis-like syndrome somewhat similar to this patient's illness. In addition rash is not uncommon in EB virus disease.

2. (B, C, D, E) A single antibody titer against the proteus OX 19 antigen greater than 1:80 is not diagnostic of rickettsial disease. As in so many serologic studies it is important to document a rise in titer during the weeks following the onset of illness. A biphasic or "saddle back" fever curve is characteristic of lymphocytic choriomeningitis as well as leptospirosis and dengue. Presumably early symptoms and signs are related to microbial invasion - late ones are likely a result of immune complex injury. Spirochetes may be grown from the urine of patients with Weils disease if appropriate media is used. Sulfonamides do appear to increase the severity of rickettsial disease. Prior to the availability of tetracycline and chloramphenicol paraamino benzoic acid was used to treat patients with rickettsial disease. Q fever is caused by Coxiella burnetii and infectious diseases caused by this rickettsia do not induce antibodies to the X strains of Proteus vulgaris. Serologic diagnosis in Q fever is made by demonstration of a titer rise against the specific antigens utilizing complement fixation or other serologic tests.

3. (A, B) The rash of murine typhus may be very evanescent and generally begins on the trunk in contrast to the rash in Rocky Mountain spotted fever where early involvement of the extremities is most common. Rats and ectoparasites of rats appear to be the major vectors for murine typhus. In the United States this illness is most commonly reported from the southeastern United States especially the Texas Gulf coast. Chloramphenicol and tetracycline are acceptable therapeutic agents for murine typhus. Most patients respond promptly in two or three days and mortality is very low in treated cases. Some reports of patients with murine typhus have demonstrated mild abnormalities of liver function as was seen here.

REFERENCES

1. Saah AJ, Hornick RB. Rickettsia typhi. Mandell GL, Douglas RG Jr, and Bennett JE, eds. Principles and Practices of Infectious Diseases. New York: John Wiley & Sons, 1979; 1523-25.

2. Gastel B (ed). Murine typhus, clinical conferences at the Johns Hopkins Hospital. Johns Hopkins Med J 1977; 141:303.

3. Older JJ. The epidemiology of murine typhus in Texas, 1969. J Am Med Assn 1970; 214:2011.

4. Stuart BM, Pullen RL. Endemic (murine) typhus fever: Clinical observations of 180 cases. Ann Intern Med 1945; 23: 520.

CASE 47

HISTORY

A 25-year-old male cattle farmer presents because of fever and malaise of three weeks' duration. He noted mild malaise and low grade fever three weeks earlier; both symptoms have become progressively worse such that at the time of presentation he becomes exhausted after two to three hours' work and has afternoon fever to 102-103°F. Two days before presentation he noted swelling and tenderness of the right scrotum.

EXAMINATION

Physical examination reveals a moderately ill man with a temperature of 102°F, mild generalized lymphadenopathy, splenomegaly and swelling and tenderness of the right testis.

LABORATORY DATA

The white blood cell count is 9,000 with 50% lymphocytes, 10% of which are atypical. Urinalysis is normal; SGOT is 150.

QUESTIONS

1. WHICH OF THE FOLLOWING IS MOST LIKELY TO BE THE CAUSE OF THIS ILLNESS?
   - A. *Brucella abortus*
   - B. Ebstein-Barr virus
   - C. *Toxoplasma gondii*
   - D. Cytomegalovirus
   - E. *Leptospira pomona*
   - F. Hepatitis virus A or B

2. BRUCELLA AGGLUTINATION TITER IS POSITIVE AT A DILUTION OF 1:1280. APPROPRIATE ANTIMICROBIAL THERAPY IS
   - A. no antimicrobial therapy
   - B. penicillin
   - C. tetracycline
   - D. streptomycin
   - E. gentamicin

3. WHICH OF THE FOLLOWING STATEMENTS IS/ARE TRUE?
   - A. Human brucellosis may be acquired from cattle, pigs, goats, and dogs
   - B. Eosinophilia is commonly seen with brucellosis
   - C. Glanders is an occupational hazard of cattle farmers in the northwestern United States

D. Most patients who develop leptospirosis have clinically apparent hepatitis and nephritis
E. The spirochete responsible for leptospirosis grows readily in routine blood culture media

ANSWERS

1. (A) Ebstein-Barr virus, Toxoplasma gondii, cytomegalovirus, hepatitis viruses, and brucellae may all cause the mononucleosis syndrome characterized by fever, atypical lymphocytosis, lymphadenopathy, and hepatitis. The patient's exposure to cattle, the duration of his illness, and especially the presence of orchitis strongly suggest that he has brucellosis.

2. (C, D) Tetracycline with or without streptomycin is appropriate treatment for brucellosis.

3. (A) Humans may acquire brucellosis from dogs as well as from cattle, pigs, and goats. Antibodies to Brucella melitensis and B. suis cross-react with B. abortus antigens, so that routine brucella agglutination determination will usually detect infection with any of these species. However, B. canis antibodies do not cross-react; so if one is suspicious of brucellosis acquired from a dog, he should obtain a B. canis titer, available at the CDC. The most commonly recognized syndrome caused by leptospiras is aseptic meningitis; the vast majority of patients infected with leptospiras do not have liver or kidney involvement. Leptospiras may be cultured from blood but only if enriched media are used.

REFERENCES

1. Hendricks SL, Borts IH, Heeren RH, et al. Brucellosis outbreak in an Iowa packing house. Am J Public Health 1962; 52:1166.

2. Buchanan TM, Faber LC, Frix MK, et al. Brucellosis in the United States, 1960-1972. An abattoir associated disease. II. Diagnostic aspects. Medicine 1974; 53:415.

3. Hall WH. Endemic brucellosis in beagles. J Infect Dis 1971; 124:615.

4. Heath CW Jr, Alexander AD, Galton MM. Leptospirosis in the United States. Analysis of 483 cases in man, 1949-1961. New Engl J Med 1965; 273:857, 915.

CASE 48

HISTORY

The Infectious Disease service is asked to see a patient with leukemia and pneumonia. He is a 36-year-old man who was admitted to the hospital one week earlier because of fever and leukopenia. Evaluation revealed acute leukemia, and treatment was begun with prednisone, cytosine arabinoside, vincristine, and daunorubicin. He was found to have a left lower lobe infiltrate. Culture of the sputum revealed many colonies of *Pseudomonas aeruginosa*, sensitive to 32 ug/ml of carbenicillin and he was treated with 24 gms of that agent per day. He responded with defervescence and remained afebrile until day of consultation.

EXAMINATION

On examination he appears acutely ill, his blood pressure is 90/50 and temperature is 104°F. Fine rales and evidence of consolidation are present over left lower lung field. The remainder of the examination is unremarkable.

LABORATORY DATA

The white blood cell count is 4,000 with 99% blast forms. Gram's stain of the sputum reveals numerous gram-negative bacilli. No other bacteria and no fungi or mycobacteria are seen on appropriately stained smears. Chest roentgenogram at this time shows progression of the pneumonia.

QUESTIONS

1. WHICH TWO OF THE FOLLOWING FORMULATIONS APPEAR MOST LIKELY AT THIS TIME?
   - A. There has been progression of the pseudomonas pneumonia due to development of resistance of the pneudomonas to carbenicillin or due to inadequate host defenses or both
   - B. The patient has *Staphylococcus aureus* superinfection
   - C. The patient has superinfection with Klebsiella resistant to carbenicillin
   - D. The patient has fungal superinfection
   - E. The patient has *Pneumocystis carinii* pneumonia

2. WHICH ONE OF THE FOLLOWING ANTIMICROBIAL AGENTS SHOULD THE PATIENT NOW RECEIVE?
   - A. Ampicillin
   - B. Cephalothin

C. Kanamycin
D. Amikacin
E. Polymyxin B

3. WHICH OF THE FOLLOWING IS/ARE TRUE?
A. Antimicrobial agents induce adaptive metabolic alterations in bacteria. Thus, the most common manner by which a bacterial population acquires resistance to a drug is by drug-induced metabolic changes
B. Conjugation is a method by which gram-negative bacilli may acquire resistance; however, this is a rare phenomenon that is not clinically important
C. Inactivation of penicillin by penicillinase-producing staphylococci present in the nasopharynx accounts for the majority of treatment failures of Group A streptococcal pharyngitis
D. The incorporation of antimicrobial agents into feed for domestic animals has resulted in increased antimicrobial resistance of many strains of Salmonella pathogenic for man

4. IN WHICH OF THE FOLLOWING SITUATIONS SHOULD PROPHYLACTIC ANTIBIOTICS BE USED?
A. Dental extraction in a patient with valvular heart disease
B. Instrumentation of the urinary tract
C. Vaginal or abdominal hysterectomy
D. Long term corticosteroid therapy in a PPD positive patient (INH)
E. Long term corticosteroid therapy in a PPD negative patient (INH)
F. Newborns to prevent ophthalmia neonatorum
G. Cardiac catheterization
H. Prolonged labor after premature rupture of membranes
I. Acute rheumatic fever

ANSWERS

1. (A, C) There have been several reports of pulmonary superinfection with Klebsiella group organisms in patients treated with carbenicillin, and this is the most likely possibility in this particular patient. In addition it is also possible that pseudomonas pneumonia might progress in spite of appropriate antimicrobial therapy in a patient with such a severe impairment of host defenses. When the absolute number of polymorphonuclear leukocytes falls below 100 per cubic millimeter, bacterial infections are very difficult to eradicate even with bactericidal chemotherapy. While staphylococcal infection is possible, it is unlikely in view of the Gram's stain. Pneumocystis

pneumonia usually presents a more diffuse pattern, and it would not be expected to begin in the exact location as the previous pseudomonas infection.

2. (D) Amikacin is the antimicrobial agent of choice in this situation because of the very real possibility of superinfection with a gram-negative organism resistant to carbenicillin. Amikacin has the widest spectrum of activity against gram-negative organisms of any presently available agent. Ticarcillin and tobramycin is a combination of drugs also of proven efficacy against Pseudomonas pneumonia in leukemic patients.

3. (D) Acquired microbial resistance to antimicrobial agents is most commonly the result of selection of resistant strains from the initial inoculum and not due to metabolic changes induced by the agent. Conjugation is actually quite important in the mediation of antimicrobial resistance among gram-negative bacilli. While it appears logical that staphylococcal penicillinase might locally decrease the effectiveness of penicillin when that agent is used to treat streptococcal pharyngitis and thereby account for treatment failures, this mechanism has in fact been disproven by careful studies.

4. (A, D, F, H, I) Because antimicrobial agents may prevent infection in some but not all surgical patients and do so with some risk, they must not be used indiscriminately. For example, prophylaxis works in vaginal but not abdominal hysterectomy. When used, antimicrobials should first be given 1-2 hours before surgery, which is enough time for therapeutic levels to be achieved but not long enough to select resistant organisms. The antimicrobial agents should usually be stopped 24 hours after surgery.

REFERENCES

1. Antimicrobial prophylaxis for surgery. Medical Letter 1979; 21:73.

2. Parry MF, New HC. A comparative study of ticarcillin plus tobramycin versus carbenicillin plus gentamicin for the treatment of serious infection due to gram-negative bacilli. Am J Med 1978; 64:961.

3. Sabath LD. Drug resistance of bacteria. New Engl J Med 1969; 280:91.

4. Watanabe T. Infectious drug resistance in enteric bacteria. New Engl J Med 1966; 275:888.

5. Lyons RW, Thornton GF, Andriole VT. Carbenicillin: Clinical and laboratory studies. J Infect Dis 1970; 122:S104.

6. Goodell B, Jacobs JB, Powell RD, DeVita VT. Pneumocystis carinii: The spectrum of diffuse interstitial pneumonia in patients with neoplastic diseases. Ann Intern Med 1970; 72: 337.

7. Quie PG, Pierce HC, Wannamaker LW. Influence of penicillinase-producing staphylococci on the erradication of group A streptococci from the upper respiratory tract by penicillin treatment. Pediatrics 1966; 37:476.

CASE 49

HISTORY

A 60-year-old woman with stage IVB Hodgkin's disease presents because of fever and headache of eight days' duration. The diagnosis of Hodgkin's disease had been made at laparotomy one year earlier. The liver, spleen, and para-aortic lymph nodes were found to be involved and the spleen was removed. She has been maintained on intermittent therapy with BACOP since that time without evidence of active disease. She became ill one week prior to the present admission with low grade fever and generalized headache. Her headache has become progressively severe and fever has been as high as 103°F. She has received no antimicrobial therapy.

EXAMINATION

Physical examination reveals a chronically ill appearing woman with nuchal rigidity, fever and a well healed, midline abdominal surgical scar. The remainder of the examination is unremarkable; no focal neurological signs are detected.

LABORATORY DATA

The hematocrit is 35%, white blood cell count 11,000 with 60% polymorphonuclear leukocytes, 6% bands, 28% lymphocytes and 6% monocytes. Platelet count is 250,000. Urinalysis, renal function, and hepatic function tests are normal. Lumbar puncture reveals an opening pressure of 240 mm; 250 white blood cells, 60% of which are mononuclear, 40% polymorphonuclear; glucose of 33 with a serum glucose of 105; and protein of 180 mg%. Gram's stain, acid fast smear, and India ink preparation do not reveal any microbial forms. Appropriate cultures are planted.

QUESTIONS

1. WHICH 4 OF THE FOLLOWING WOULD YOU MOST SERIOUSLY CONSIDER AS THE CAUSE OF HER ILLNESS?
   - A. *Listeria monocytogenes* meningitis
   - B. *Cryptococcus neoformans* meningitis
   - C. *Staphylococcus aureus* meningitis
   - D. *Hemophilus influenzae* meningitis
   - E. *Streptococcus pneumoniae* meningitis
   - F. Brain abscess
   - G. Infiltration of the meninges by lymphoma cells
   - H. *Mycobacterium tuberculosis* meningitis

I. Coxsackie virus meningitis
J. Herpes simplex encephalitis
K. Leptospiral meningitis

2. BASED UPON THE ABOVE RESULTS, YOU WOULD IMMEDIATELY BEGIN TREATMENT WITH
A. amphotericin B intravenously
B. penicillin G 20,000,000 units intravenously daily
C. ampicillin 12 gm intravenously daily
D. chloramphenicol 4-6 gm intravenously daily
E. gentamicin 5 mg/kg intravenously daily and 5 mg intrathecally daily
F. 5 fluorocytosine 150 mg/kg/day by mouth
G. isoniazid and rifampin in appropriate doses
H. intrathecal methotrexate
I. none of the above

Two days later the following information is available: Bacteriologic culture of the cerebrospinal fluid has revealed a beta hemolytic pleomorphic gram-positive bacillus. Cryptococcal antigen determination is negative. Cerebrospinal fluid cytologic examination reveals no abnormal cells. PPD and mumps skin tests are negative.

3. YOUR INTERPRETATION OF THESE RESULTS IS
A. the bacterium isolated is probably a skin contaminant
B. laboratory personnel should perform biochemical tests to further define the isolate
C. the isolate is likely a species of clostridia
D. the report of the Gram's stain of the isolate is probably in error; the microorganism is probably _Streptococcus pneumoniae_
E. acid fast smear of the isolate will probably be positive

ANSWERS

1. (A, B, G, H) The patient has impaired cell mediated immunity and is therefore susceptible to infection with opportunistic bacteria and fungi. The clinical presentation of a subacute illness and the CSF findings argue strongly against meningitis due to a pyogenic bacterium. The depressed CSF glucose argues against viral and leptospiral meningitis and encephalitis, and the absence of focal findings and low CSF glucose argue against brain abscess. Listeria, cryptococcus, tuberculosis, and infiltration of the meninges with lymphoma cells are all consistent with her clinical course and the CSF findings.

2. (C, G) Any patient with lymphocytic meningitis associated with low CSF glucose should be treated initially for tuberculous meningitis. We would include treatment for listeria as well in this immunocompromised patient. While cryptococcal meningitis is certainly possible, we would not treat her with amphotericin B initially but would obtain a cryptococcal antigen determination on the CSF.

3. (B) As indicated above, in this clinical setting the isolate is very likely to be Listeria monocytogenes. Since the isolation of diphtheroids from clinical specimens usually results from contamination of the culture by skin flora, most microbiology laboratories discard these isolates as contaminants. It is critically important in a case such as this one that the physician alert the laboratory to the possibility that the "diphtheroid" may be listeria and ask that they further define the isolate and perform antimicrobial susceptibility testing.

REFERENCES

1. Chernik NL, Armstrong D, Posner JB. Central nervous system infections in patients with cancer. Medicine 1974; 52: 563.

2. Smith HV. Tuberculous meningitis. Internatl J Neurol 1964; 4:134.

3. Buchanan RE, Gibbon NE. Bergey's Manual of Determinative Bacteriology. Baltimore: Williams and Wilkins, Co., 1974; 593-596.

4. Lavetter A, Leedom JM, Mathies AW, et al. Meningitis due to Listeria monocytogenes. A review of 25 cases. New Engl J Med 1971; 285:598.

5. Medoff G, Kunz LJ, Weinberg AN. Listeriosis in humans: an evaluation. J Infect Dis 1971; 123:247.

CASE 50

HISTORY

A 27-year-old man presents to the emergency room with the chief complaint of cough and fever of two days' duration. Two days previously he noted the onset of weakness and malaise and retired early. Early the next morning he had a shaking chill which lasted 15 minutes. When he took his temperature one hour later, it was 103°F. Several hours later he noted the onset of right lower chest pain, which was aggravated by taking a deep breath and by coughing. That evening his cough became productive of "rusty" sputum. All the symptoms progressed until the time of his presentation to the emergency room. There were no subsequent chills.

EXAMINATION

Physical examination reveals an acutely ill young man with normal blood pressure, pulse rate of 120, respiratory rate of 32, and temperature of 103°F. Positive findings are slightly cyanotic lips and nail beds; splinting of the right chest; and increased fremitus, dullness, and fine inspiratory rales over the right lateral chest.

LABORATORY DATA

Gram's stain of the sputum reveals many polymorphonuclear leukocytes and gram-positive diplococci. The chest roentgenogram reveals consolidation of the right lower lobe.

QUESTIONS

1. THE MICROORGANISM WHICH IS MOST LIKELY RESPONSIBLE FOR THIS ILLNESS IS
   - A. *Staphylococcus aureus*
   - B. *Mycoplasma pneumoniae*
   - C. *Klebsiella pneumoniae*
   - D. *Streptococcus pneumoniae*
   - E. adenovirus, type 4

Twenty-four hours following the initiation of appropriate antimicrobial therapy the patient becomes afebrile and remains so until five days later when he is once again noted to have fever, this time 101°F. Physical examination reveals little change in the lungs; however, the roentgenogram shows partial clearing of the previously noted infiltrate. The patient states that he is feeling better each day.

2. THE MOST LIKELY CAUSE OF RECURRENT FEVER IS
   A. bacterial superinfection, e.g. gram-negative bacillary pneumonia
   B. lung abscess
   C. drug fever
   D. bronchial obstruction
   E. relapse of pneumoncoccal pneumonia due to the development of resistance of the organism to penicillin G

3. WHICH OF THE FOLLOWING STATEMENTS IS/ARE TRUE?
   A. Proteinuria and hyponatremia are well recognized complications of pneumococcal pneumonia
   B. The finding of hyperbilirubinemia in the patient presented would militate against the diagnosis of pneumococcal pneumonia
   C. Empyema and pneumothorax are fairly frequent complications of staphylococcal pneumonia in children
   D. The development of decreased or absent tactile fremitus over the right lower chest in the patient presented would be consistent with uncomplicated resolving pneumococcal pneumonia
   E. Pneumococcal vaccine (Pneumovax^{R}) is effective in preventing pneumococcal pneumonia
   F. Pneumovax contains live attenuated bacteria

ANSWERS

1. (D) This is a fairly typical case of pneumococcal pneumonia.

2. (C) The improving general condition of the patient and the clearing noted on the roentgenogram militate strongly against the presence of pulmonary superinfection, lung abscess or relapse. In addition, pneumococci rarely develop resistance to penicillin G. It is important to emphasize, however, than any patient who develops fever while being treated for one variety of bacterial pneumonia should be carefully evaluated for the possibilities listed.

3. (A, C, E) Hyperbilirubinemia is in fact fairly common in patients with moderate to severe pneumococcal pneumonia. The development of decreased or absent tactile fremitus implies effusion, bronchial obstruction or empyema. Each is a complication of pneumococcal pneumonia.

REFERENCES

1. Wood WB. Pneumococcal pneumonia. In: Beeson PB, McDermott W. Textbook of Medicine. Philadelphia: WB Saunders Co., 1967; 145-159.

2. Austrian R, Gold J. Pneumococcal bacteremia with especial reference to bacteremic pneumococcal pneumonia. Ann Intern Med 1964; 60:759.

3. Hansman D, Glascow H, Sturt J, et al. Increased resistance to penicillin of pneumococci isolated from man. New Engl J Med 1971; 284:175.

4. Pneumococcal vaccine. Medical Letter 1978; 20:13.

CASE 51

HISTORY

A 23-year-old white woman in her 35th week of pregnancy was admitted to the hospital for treatment of toxemia of pregnancy. Three days after admission the absence of fetal heart tones was detected, and she was delivered of a dead fetus. It is now four days later, and she has become confused, jaundiced, febrile, and oliguric.

EXAMINATION

On physical examination the patient is an acutely ill, jaundiced woman. Her BP is 90/40, pulse rate 128, temperature 103.6° F, and respirations 26. Her skin is cold and clammy. The sclerae are icteric. There is diffuse abdominal tenderness especially in the supra-pubic area. Pelvic examination reveals an enlarged boggy, tender uterus, and a serosanguineous cervical discharge.

LABORATORY DATA

Laboratory data include a hematocrit of 17% and a WBC count of 34,000 with a marked "shift to the left". There are nucleated RBC's and erythrophagocytosis noted on peripheral smear. The urine gives a 4+ hemoglobulin reaction and is wine-colored. The indirect bilirubin is 19 mgm% with a total of 23. An abdominal film shows gas in the uterus.

QUESTIONS

1. BLOOD CULTURES WILL PROBABLY REVEAL
   A. Leptospira icto-hemorrhagiaca
   B. Clostridium perfringens
   C. Bacteriodes species
   D. E. coli
   E. Staphylococcus aureus

2. APPROPRIATE MANAGEMENT WOULD INCLUDE
   A. parenteral antibiotics, to include penicillin and chloramphenicol
   B. total abdominal hysterectomy
   C. polyvalent clostridial antitoxin
   D. Gram's stain of the cervical discharge
   E. leptospiral agglutinins

3. WHICH OF THE FOLLOWING ORGANISMS ARE COMMONLY RECOVERED FROM PATIENTS WITH SEPTIC ABORTION?

A. *Clostridium perfringens*
B. *Bacteroides sp.*
C. *Staphylococcus aureus*
D. *E. coli*
E. Anaerobic *streptococcus* (*Peptostreptococcus*)

4. WHICH OF THE FOLLOWING DISORDERS ARE CAUSED BY *CLOSTRIDIUM* SPECIES?

A. Tetanus
B. Botulism
C. Food poisoning
D. Pseudomembranous enterocolitis
E. Anthrax

ANSWERS

1. (B) The case described is a typical example of uterine myonecrosis caused by *Clostridium perfringens*. Hemolysis results from a lecithinase elaborated by the organism and produces hemoglobinuria with jaundice and renal failure. The disorder usually begins 2-3 days after a septic abortion, but occasionally may follow a normal delivery.

2. (A, B, C, D) Parenteral antibiotics should be directed against aerobic gram-negative bacilli as well as anaerobes. Penicillin and chloramphenicol or clindamycin and an aminoglycoside are the usual regimens. Currettage may avoid hysterectomy in less severe cases, but when extensive invasion of the uterus and adjacent structures is associated with bacteremia and hemolysis, hysterectomy is usually required. Although polyvalent clostridial antitoxin is of questionable value, in patients with uterine myonecrosis and "septico-toxemia" its use is wise.

3. (E) Fulminant *Clostridium perfringens* infection of the type demonstrated by this case is fortunately rare, accounting for less than 1% of post-abortal sepsis. Anaerobes, including *Bacteroides* and *Peptostreptococcus*, and aerobic gram-negative bacilli are the common pathogens.

4. (A, B, C, D) Clostridial enterotoxin causes acute diarrheal food poisoning. The toxin elaborated by *Clostridium difficile* causes pseudomembraneous enterocolitis.

REFERENCES

1. Decker WH, Hall W. Treatment of abortions infected with *Clostridium welchii*. Am J Obstet Gynecol 1966; 95:394.

2. Patchell RD. Clostridial myonecrosis of the postpartum uterus with radiologic diagnosis. Obstet Gynecol 1978; 51S:14.

3. Eaton CJ, Peterson EP. Diagnosis and acute management of patients with advanced clostridial sepsis complicating abortion. Am J Obstet Gynecol 1971; 109:1162.

4. Rotheram EB, Schick SF. Non-clostridial anaerobic bacteremia in septic abortion. Am J Med 1969; 46:80.

5. Smith JW, Southern PM, Lehmann JD. Bacteremia in septic abortion. Complications and treatment. Obstet Gynecol 1970; 35:704.

CASE 52

HISTORY

A 40-year-old physician's wife sought medical attention because of an infected bite. Two days previously, she had attempted to separate the combatants in a dog fight and had been bitten on the left thigh. She cleansed the wound with soap and water; however, two days later, she noted soreness, redness and a watery discharge. There was no history of any prior health problem.

EXAMINATION

Physical examination was unremarkable except for the wound which appeared inflamed and was tender. Gram stain of the discharge revealed moderate numbers of polymorphonuclear leukocytes and a few gram-positive and gram-negative forms. Because of a clinical suspicion of either staphylococcal or group A streptococcal cellulitis, oral cloxacillin was prescribed following culture of the lesion. Twenty-four hours later there had been no improvement and the culture revealed what appeared to be streptococcal colonies on the blood agar plate. There was no growth on the EMB plate. Gram stain of a colony smear showed small pleomorphic gram-negative bacilli.

QUESTIONS

1. WHICH OF THE FOLLOWING STATEMENTS REGARDING THIS PATIENT IS/ARE TRUE?
   - A. The culture results are probably misleading and the etiologic bacterium is most likely group A streptococcus or _Staphylococcus aureus_
   - B. This probably represents _Haemophilus influenzae_ cellulitis
   - C. _Pasteurella multocida_ is a likely etiologic microorganism
   - D. Mixed aerobic and anaerobic bacilli are probably responsible
   - E. Prior splenectomy might have increased the risk of more serious disease

The culture is identified on the next day as _Pasteurella multocida_.

2. WHICH OF THE FOLLOWING STATEMENTS ABOUT THIS BACTERIUM IS/ARE TRUE?
   - A. _Pasteurella multocida_ is a frequent inhabitant of the oral cavity of healthy dogs and cats
   - B. It is the most common bacterium identified in infected dog bites

C. Pasteurella multocida is commonly recovered from infected human bites
D. Pasteurella multocida has been reported to cause meningitis, arthritis, and pleuropulmonary disease as well as dog and cat bite infections

3. WHICH OF THE FOLLOWING ANTIMICROBIAL AGENTS IS APPROPRIATE THERAPY FOR PASTEURELLA MULTOCIDA INFECTION?
A. Penicillinase-resistant penicillins, i.e. nafcillin, cloxacillin
B. Penicillin G
C. Tetracycline
D. Parenteral vancomycin
E. Oral chloramphenicol

ANSWERS

1. (C, E) The recovery of small pleomorphic gram-negative bacilli from an infected dog or cat bite strongly suggests Pasteurella multocida as the etiology. Haemophilus influenzae may cause cellulitis, especially in the cervical and thoracic area, but is very uncommon in the situation described. A "new" microorganism, DF-2, may cause fatal disease in splenectomized patients following dog bite.

2. (A, B, D) Pasteurella multocida has been recovered from the oral pharynx of a number of animals, including cattle, horses, swine, sheep, fowl, dogs, cats, and rats. Cat scratch fever, staphylococcal and streptococcal cellulitis and tularemia should also be considered in an infected bite. Pasteurella multocida is rarely recovered from infected human bites. In that situation a variety of bacteria may be recovered. Recent reports suggest that anaerobic species were present in at least half of infected human bites, bacteroides and fusobacterium being most common. Pasteurella multocida has been reported to cause a variety of other clinical infectious disease disorders. They include pleuro-pulmonary disease, bacteremia, arthritis and meningitis.

3. (B, C) Penicillin G is the antimicrobial agent of choice for Pasteurella multocida infection.

REFERENCES

1. Johnson RH, Rumans LW. Unusual infections caused by Pasteurella multocida. J Am Med Assn 1977; 237:146.

2. Francis DP, Holmes MA, Brandon G. Pasteurella multocida. Infections after domestic animal bites and scratches. J Am Med Assn 1975; 233:42.

3. Goldstein EJC, Caffee HH, Price JE, et al. Human bite infections. Lancet 1977; 1290.

4. Bailie WE, Stowe EC, Schmitt AM. Aerobic bacterial flora of oral and nasal fluids of canines with reference to bacteria associated with bites. J Clin Micro 1978; 2:223.

5. Check W. An odd link between dog bites, splenectomy. J Am Med Assn 1979; 241:225.

CASE 53

HISTORY

This was the first University Hospital admission for this 67-year-old man who was transferred from another hospital for management of hemoptysis. Ten years earlier, because of aortic stenosis, the patient's aortic valve was replaced by a Starr Edwards prosthetic device and he had taken Coumadin since. Pulmonary tuberculosis was diagnosed one year prior to admission and the patient given isoniazid and ethambutol. Three months later because of the appearance of hepatitis isoniazid was discontinued. Liver biopsy revealed chronic, aggressive hepatitis and corticosteroid therapy was begun. Two weeks prior to admission the chest roentgenogram was noted to have worsened, there were large cavities and more evidence of inflammatory change. One week prior to admission hemoptysis began and he was admitted to another hospital. On the day of transfer massive hemoptysis occurred.

EXAMINATION

On admission to University Hospital, the physical examination revealed an anxious, mildly hypotensive man, coughing up large quantities of bright, red blood. There were a few scattered rales bilaterally in the apices and heart sounds were characteristic of a normally functioning prosthetic aortic valve.

LABORATORY DATA

Laboratory evaluation revealed a normal hemogram. The serum SGOT was 85 IU, the alkaline phosphatase 150 IU and the Hb_sAg was positive.

QUESTIONS

1. WHICH OF THE FOLLOWING STATEMENTS CONCERNING PULMONARY TUBERCULOSIS IS/ARE TRUE?
   - A. In a patient with presumed inactive pulmonary tuberculosis hemoptysis suggests reactivation
   - B. Most patients with chronic cavitary pulmonary tuberculosis become ill soon, e.g. within six months, after initial exposure to the etiologic mycobacteria
   - C. As many as 25% of patients with active pulmonary tuberculosis will have negative skin tests with intermediate PPD at the time the illness is first diagnosed

D. Patients with active pulmonary tuberculosis, whose sputum contains viable acid fast organisms, may become significantly less infective within days after initiation of appropriate antimicrobial therapy
E. Patients on hemodialysis and patients with ileal bypass procedures for obesity appear to be at increased risk of development of active tuberculosis

2. WHICH OF THE FOLLOWING STATEMENTS CONCERNING ISONIAZID INDUCED HEPATITIS IS/ARE CORRECT?
A. Isoniazid induced hepatitis can be distinguished from acute viral hepatitis by careful examination of a liver biopsy sample
B. Patients who are rapid acetylators of isoniazid develop hepatotoxicity more frequently than slow acetylators
C. A metabolic product of isoniazid, acetyl hydrazine, may be responsible for hepatotoxicity

3. WHICH OF THE FOLLOWING STATEMENTS REGARDING TUBERCULOSIS THERAPY IS/ARE CORRECT?
A. Rifampin is contraindicated in patients with prior hepatitis caused by isoniazid
B. Rifampin may cause reversible acute renal failure associated with light chain proteinuria
C. Ethambutol alone is appropriate prophylaxis for patients who are allergic to isoniazid
D. Corticosteroid therapy of patients with positive tuberculin skin tests clearly increases the risk of subsequent development of active disease and is an indication for isoniazid prophylaxis
E. Short-course therapy is an acceptible substitute for some patients with pulmonary tuberculosis

ANSWERS

1. (A, C, D, E) Hemoptysis usually indicates reactivation of pulmonary tuberculosis. Erosion of bronchial vessels, and Rassmusen aneurysms are found in pathologic specimens from the lungs of such patients. Generally, cavitary pulmonary tuberculosis is a result of tissue destruction by tuberculous microorganisms which have been present for a long duration, often years. When pulmonary tuberculosis follows soon after initial infection, the pneumonic infiltrates tend to involve lower lobes and pleura (tuberculous pneumonia). The intermediate PPD is not always positive in patients with active pulmonary tuberculosis. This may be due to relative or absolute anergy in debilitated patients and/or poor skin test antigen placement either due to technique or lack of subcutaneous tissue. Several

studies have suggested patients with active pulmonary tuberculosis are less infective even after a brief period of antimicrobial therapy. For this reason, early hospital discharge is probably appropriate when proper therapy has been selected. There appears to be an increased susceptibility to tuberculosis among patients with ileal bypass procedures or on chronic hemodialysis. Presumably, each of these conditions interferes in some way with delayed type hypersensitivity thereby increasing susceptibility to clinical disease.

2. (B, C) Hepatitis caused by isoniazid is indistinguishable from acute viral hepatitis. Rapid acetylators appear to be more susceptible to hepatotoxicity. Acetyl hydrazine and other metabolic products of isoniazid may be responsible for hepatotoxicity. Patients who are rapid acetylators may have a higher risk of liver disease because they produce more of these metabolites.

3. (B, E) Rifampin is not absolutely contraindicated in patients with prior hepatitis caused by isoniazid although the risk of additional damage is probably greater than in the patient who has had no prior difficulty. The agents are chemically dissimilar and there is no evidence of cross allergenicity. Rifampin has been reported to cause light chain proteinuria and reversible renal insufficiency. There have been no studies which demonstrate effective prophylaxis of tuberculous disease by any agent other than isoniazid. Prophylaxis for patients with a positive skin test who are to receive corticosteroid therapy is debatable. One study in patients receiving corticosteroids for bronchial asthma suggested patients with positive PPDs were at no greater risk than those with negative PPDs and advised against routine isoniazid prophylaxis. A recent report summarizes guidelines for short-course anti-tuberculous therapy. They include the recommendation of a "core" of INH and rifampin for a minimum of 9 months with daily initial therapy for 2 weeks to 2 months and follow up for 12 months after completion of treatment.

REFERENCES

1. Current trends: Preventative therapy of tuberculous infection. Morbidity and Mortality Weekly Report 1975; February: 71.

2. Mitchell JR, Zimmerman HJ, Ishak KG, et al. Isoniazid liver injury: Clinical spectrum, pathology, and probable pathogenesis. Ann Int Med 1976; 84:181.

3. Schatz M, Patterson R, Kloner R, Falk J. The prevalence of tuberculosis and positive tuberculin skin tests in a steroid-treated asthmatic population. Ann Int Med 1976; 84:261.

4. Nelson SD, Mitchell JR, Timbrell JA, Snodgrass WR, Corcoran GB III. Isoniazid and Iproniazid: Activation of metabolites to toxic intermediates in man and rat. Science 1976; 193:901.

5. Kumar S, Mehta JA, Trivedi HL. Communications to the editor: Light-chain proteinuria and reversible renal failure in rifampin-treated patients with tuberculosis. Chest 1976; 70: 564.

6. Andrew OT, Schoenfeld PY, Howewell PC, Humphreys MH. Tuberculosis in patients with end-stage renal disease. Am J Med 1980; 68:59.

7. Rutsky EA, Rostand SG. Mycobacteriosis in patients with chronic renal failure. Arch Int Med 1979; 140:57.

8. Current Trends: Guidelines for short-course tuberculosis chemotherapy. Morbidity and Mortality Weekly Report 1980; 29:97.

CASE 54

HISTORY

A 30-year-old man with aortic valvular incompetence has enterococcal endocarditis. Five years previously he developed a macular, erythematous rash one week following treatment with penicillin G. He did not have urticaria, wheezing, dyspnea or faintness at that time. He has received no penicillin since then. Skin tests with benzylpenicilloyl -polylysine (BPL) and a "minor determinant mixture" (MDM) are negative.

QUESTIONS

1. HIS SERUM WOULD PROBABLY CONTAIN DETECTABLE TITERS OF PENICILLIN ANTIBODY AMONG WHICH OF THE FOLLOWING CLASSES?
   A. IgG
   B. IgE
   C. IgM
   D. IgA
   E. None of the above

2. THE PATIENT IS TREATED WITH PENICILLIN G. ON THE SECOND DAY HE HAS AN URTICARIAL REACTION. IF PENICILLIN IS CONTINUED, WHICH OF THE FOLLOWING IS THE MOST LIKELY RESULT?
   A. He will continue to have urticaria until the drug is stopped
   B. He will probably have an anaphylactic reaction at some time during the course of treatment
   C. Urticaria will disappear within 2-4 days and not recur
   D. He will subsequently develop Coombs positive hemolytic anemia
   E. Urticaria will disappear only if the dose of penicillin is lowered

3. WHICH OF THE FOLLOWING IS/ARE TRUE?
   A. The immunoglobulin class most often responsible for immediate anaphylactic reactions, e.g. hypotension, urticaria, laryngeal edema and bronchospasm, is IgG.
   B. The immunoglobulin class most often responsible for immediate anaphylactic reactions, e.g. hypotension, urticaria, laryngeal edema and bronchospasm, is IgE.
   C. The process of desensitization is actually one of inducing "blocking antibody" which competes successfully for penicillin binding sites and prevents penicillin binding to IgE

D. Penicillin per se is antigenic.
E. Skin testing with BPL and MDM allows one to predict which patients will have a morbilliform rash if given penicillin

ANSWERS

1. (C) Low titers of penicillin antibodies of the IgM class are seen in approximately 98% of people in the United States. This is probably because of previous exposure to this agent. Antibodies among the other immunoglobulin classes are not generally detectable.

2. (C) The proposed mechanism for the disappearance of the skin rash is as follows: The urticarial rash is mediated by substances, e.g. histamine, elaborated by mast cells when penicillin binds to anti-penicillin IgE on the mast cell surface. With continuation of penicillin there is production of anti-penicillin IgG, which binds to penicillin and prevents its binding to anti-penicillin IgE antibodies in tissue.

3. (B, C) The mechanism most often responsible for anaphylaxis is the binding of antigen to mast cell-bound IgE, as described above. However, IgG-antigen complexes can also cause anaphylaxis. Here, the immune complexes fix complement, generating all of the complement mediators, including the anaphylatoxin C3a. C3a can bind to the mast cell surface, independent of IgE, and trigger the release of vasoactive amines. Penicillin is a hapten and must bind to serum protein in order to be antigenic. Skin testing with the benzylpenicilloyl-polylysine skin test antigen and with the minor determinant mixture allows one to predict with some degree of confidence patients who will not have an immediate allergic reaction if given penicillin. Skin testing does not allow one to identify persons who will have delayed skin rashes.

REFERENCES

1. Levine BB. Immunologic mechanisms of penicillin allergy: A haptenic model system for the study of allergic diseases of man. New Engl J Med 1966; 275:1115.

2. Levine BB, Zolov DM. Prediction of penicillin allergy by immunological tests. J Allergy 1969; 43:231.

CASE 55

HISTORY

A 27-year-old white male presented to his private physician because of headache and fever of two weeks duration. Five years previously he had moved from Alabama to Arizona and had worked there in a copper mine. Six months previously, while still living in Arizona he noted the onset of headache and low grade fever which caused him to seek medical attention.

EXAMINATION

Physical examination then was normal except for mild nuchal rigidity, but lumbar puncture revealed a lymphocytic pleocytosis with mildly depressed spinal fluid glucose.

QUESTIONS

1. THE DIFFERENTIAL DIAGNOSIS OF THIS PATIENTS' ILLNESS SHOULD INCLUDE
    - A. tuberculosis meningitis
    - B. cryptococcal meningitis
    - C. carcinomatous meningitis
    - D. herpesvirus hominis encephalitis
    - E. coccidioidal meningitis

Spinal fluid examination revealed complement fixing antibodies directed against coccidioidin at a titer of 1:8. Therapy for coccidioidal meningitis was initiated.

2. THERAPY FOR COCCIDIOIDAL MENINGITIS SHOULD INCLUDE
    - A. transfer factor
    - B. parenteral amphotericin B
    - C. interferon
    - D. intrathecal, intraventricular or intracisternal amphotericin B
    - E. rifampin
    - F. miconazole

The patient was treated with three times weekly intracisternal therapy with amphotericin B followed by two times weekly and then one time weekly therapy for a total duration of three months. The patient did well following discontinuation of therapy until the two weeks prior to presentation in Alabama when headache and fever returned. Repeat LP at this time again revealed lymphocytic pleocytosis and a complement fixing antibody titer of 1:4 against coccidioidin.

3. THERAPY AT THIS TIME SHOULD INCLUDE
   A. no therapy until Coccidioidis immitis is grown from spinal fluid
   B. prompt reinitiation of therapy including intracisternal and parenteral therapy with amphotericin B
   C. ventriculo-atrial shunt even though the spinal fluid pressure is not presently elevated
   D. radiation to the cranium
   E. placement of an Ommaya reservoir into the cisternal area for ease of delivery of amphotericin to the basal meninges

ANSWERS

1. (A, B, C, E,) Unless an etiologic microorganism or malignant cells are detected in the cerebrospinal fluid early on it is impossible to distinguish infectious meningitis from carcinomatous meningitis. Tubercule bacilli are uncommonly observed in cerebrospinal fluid of patients with tuberculosis meningitis although cultures of spinal fluid may be positive in as many as 40 to 50% of patients. Approximately one half of patients with cryptococcal meningitis will have a positive India Ink preparation when they present. Cryptococcal antigen is almost always present in cerebrospinal fluid of patients with this disorder. Coccidioidomycosis occurs only in patients who have lived in the endemic area or have been exposed to fomites, such as cotton, fruit, etc. from an endemic area. Herpesvirus hominus type 1 may cause a meningo-encephalitis in adults and the type II agent may cause aseptic meningitis in association with genital herpes disease, however neither one of these is very likely in this patient with subacute lymphocytic meningitis. Miconazole probably is not effective therapy for coccidioidomycosis of the central nervous system - some early favorable reports not withstanding.

2. (B, D) "Transfer factor" an extract of disrupted leukocytes with a molecular weight of approximately 10,000 daltons has been administered to some patients with severe coccidioidomycosis, however there is presently no convincing evidence that this has significantly changed their outcome and it is presently not being used in patients with coccidioidal meningitis. Parenteral amphotericin B along with drug delivered directly to the subarachnoid space is the therapy of choice for coccidioidal meningitis. It probably is most reasonable to try and deliver the amphotericin directly into the cisterna magna since the most extensive pathologic changes are found in the basal meninges. Since prolonged therapy is often required, arachnoiditis is a serious problem with repeated intrathecal inoculations of

amphotericin B. Intraventricular amphotericin may not deliver the drug to the site of disease as well as intracisternal therapy. Interferon, which may have a role in treatment of viral disorders as well as malignant disease, is of no value in patients with disseminated fungal infection, nor has rifampin been shown to be helpful in coccidioidal meningitis.

3. (B, E) The physician should not wait for Coccidioides immitis to grow from spinal fluid before initiating therapy for coccidioidal meningitis. Cultures are positive in only about one third of patients and visualization of the spherule form is extremely uncommon. A persistently elevated complement fixing titer against coccidioidin along with a clinical syndrome consistent with coccidioidal meningitis is sufficient evidence to justify initiation of therapy. Parenteral as well as cisternal therapy is optimal as mentioned above. Ventriculo-atrial shunts may be necessary for patients with communicating or noncommunicating hydrocephalus however they should not be done prophylactically and would not be indicated at present in this patient. Radiation to the cranium is inappropriate. An Ommaya reservoir was placed into the cisterna magna on this patient and has allowed easier delivery of drug to the basal meninges.

REFERENCES

1. Stevens DA. Coccidioides immitis. In: Mandell GL, Douglas RG Jr, and Bennett JE, eds. Principles and Practices of Infectious Diseases. New York: John Wiley & Sons, 1979; 2053-66.

2. Deresinski SC. Coccidioidomycosis in compromised hosts - experience at Stanford University Hospital. Medicine 1975; 54:377.

3. Drutz DJ, Catanzaro A. Coccidioidomycosis. Am Rev Resp Dis 1978; 117:559.

4. Meyer RD, Sattler FR, Linne SR, Ruskin J. Miconazole for treatment of disseminated coccidioidomycosis - unfavorable experience. Chest 1978; 73:825.

5. Steele RW. Therapy for disseminated coccidioidomycosis with transfer factor from a related donor. Am J Med 1976; 61:283.

CASE 56

HISTORY

A 15-year-old boy is admitted to the hospital because of burns involving 50% of his body surface area

QUESTIONS

1. INITIAL ANTIMICROBIAL THERAPY SHOULD INCLUDE
   - A. topical antibacterial creams to decrease colonization of the burn surfaces
   - B. a systemic antimicrobial agent directed against the group A beta hemolytic streptococcus
   - C. broad spectrum antibacterial coverage against staphylococcus and aerobic gram-negative bacilli
   - D. topical amphotericin B
   - E. tetanus prophylaxis

2. WHICH OF THE FOLLOWING STATEMENTS ABOUT HOST DEFENSE FACTORS IN BURNED PATIENTS IS/ARE TRUE?
   - A. Polymorphonuclear leukocytes from patients with severe burns demonstrate quantitative defects in ability to kill ingested bacteria
   - B. Serum immunoglobulin levels remain depressed in patients with burns and predispose to bacterial infection
   - C. There appears to be a defect in the inflammatory response in the subcutaneous tissue of patients with serious burns, leading to a disorder called "burn wound sepsis"
   - D. Reticuloendothelial system function is characteristically abnormal in burn patients

3. WHICH OF THE FOLLOWING STATEMENTS ABOUT BACTERIAL INFECTION IN PATIENTS WITH BURNS IS/ARE TRUE?
   - A. Active immunization with polyvalent pseudomonas vaccine has been reported to decrease the mortality from pseudomonas infection
   - B. Some burn patients appear to have increased glomerular filtration which results in inadequate serum levels of aminoglycoside antimicrobial agents if the usual dosages are employed
   - C. In many large medical centers strains of *Pseudomonas aeruginosa* are more likely to be susceptible to tobramycin than to gentamicin

Ten days following admission, the patient's temperature continues to spike to 104°F and he appears more ill. One day later the laboratory reports that *Staphylococcus aureus* is growing from all 4 blood cultures obtained during the previous three days.

4. WHICH OF THE FOLLOWING COURSES OF ACTION IS/ ARE APPROPRIATE AT THIS TIME?
   A. Removal of indwelling intravenous devices followed by additional blood cultures
   B. Initiation of parenteral anti-staphylococcal therapy
   C. Repeat physical examination looking especially for sites of metastatic staphylococcal localization such as the central nervous system, lung, heart, and kidneys.

ANSWERS

1. (A, B, E) Antibacterial creams containing mafenide acetate (Sulfamylon), 0.5% silver nitrate or silver sulfadiazine have been demonstrated to decrease the likelihood of serious infection in patients with burns. Most burn centers employ low dose penicillin therapy for all patients admitted with burns to prevent group A beta hemolytic streptococcal cellulitis. Broad spectrum antimicrobial agents are not indicated for initial therapy of patients with burns since they only hasten colonization by resistant microorganisms. Topical amphotericin B is of no use in such situations. Tetanus prophylaxis is necessary.

2. (A, C) Several studies have shown decreased intracellular killing by polymorphonuclear leukocytes from patients with severe burns. While there may be a transient decrease in immunoglobulin concentrations initially, later serum immunoglobulin levels are actually elevated. There does appear to be a defect in the inflammatory response in the subcutaneous tissue of patients with severe burns and infection of this area has been called burn wound sepsis. There is no discernable defect in reticuloendothelial system function in patients with burns.

3. (A, B, C) Several trials in experimental animals and a few trials in man have appeared to demonstrate the efficacy of active immunization against *Pseudomonas aeruginosa*. The report by Jones et al, is especially noteworthy. Loirat et al, reported studies which demonstrated increased glomerular filtration rate in some patients with burns. This supra-normal renal function resulted in increased clearance of aminoglycoside antimicrobial agents and necessitated larger dosages. A number of investigators from large medical centers have observed tobramycin to be slightly more active than gentamicin against strains of *Pseudomonas aeruginosa*. On the other hand in many community hospitals, where *Pseudomonas aeruginosa* disease is unusual,

most all isolates of this bacteria are still susceptible to gentamicin. At our hospital, when life-threatening Pseudomonas aeruginosa disease is suspected, we presently initiate therapy with tobramycin.

4. (A, B, C) Recovery of Staphylococcus aureus from the blood on three different days is evidence for sustained staphylococcal bacteremia and necessitates parenteral antistaphyloccal therapy. A recent report from the University of Cincinnati College of Medicine compares current patterns of staphylococcal bacteremia with the classic report of Wilson and Hamburger from the same institution. In the earlier study infective endocarditis complicated staphylococcal bacteremia in 64% of patients, whereas in the recent report it occurred in only 16%. The decreased incidence of underlying rheumatic valvular disease as well as the frequency nowdays of catheter induced bacteremia probably accounted for some of the difference. It is unclear precisely how long patients with staphylococcal bacteremia need be treated especially when the disease follows local infection at a removable site. Several studies are presently underway addressing the problem. In the present patient, if blood cultures remain positive following removal of the intravenous device, the duration of therapy probably should be at least four weeks.

REFERENCES

1. Anderson EL, Gramling PK, Vestal PR, Farrar WE Jr. Susceptibility of Pseudomonas aeruginosa to tobramycin or gentamicin alone and combined with carbenicillin. Antimicrob Agents Chemother 1975; 8:300.

2. Burke JF. Burns. In: Mandell GL, Douglas RG Jr, and Bennett JE, eds. Principles and Practices of Infectious Diseases. New York: John Wiley & Sons, 1979; 838-43.

3. Feller I, Flora JD Jr, Bawol R. Baseline results of therapy for burned patients. J Am Med Assn 1976; 236(17):1943.

4. Jones RJ, Roe EA, Gupta JL. Low mortality in burned patients in a Pseudomonas vaccine trial. Lancet, August 19, 1978; 401-03

5. Loirat P, Roham J, Baillet A, et al. Increased glomerular filtration rate in patients with major burns and its effect on the pharmacokinetics of tobramycin. N Engl J Med 1978; 299: 915.

6. Shah M, Watanakunakorn C. Changing patterns of *Staphylococcus aureus* bacteremia. Am J Med Sci 1979; 278:115.

CASE 57

HISTORY

A 13-year-old white boy who lives in Nigeria with his missionary parents is admitted to the hospital because of a six-hour history of chills, fever, and right flank pain accompanied by frequency and dysuria. He has not had a similar illness before, although he has had intermittent hematuria.

EXAMINATION

On physical examination he is found to have a temperature of 104°F, blood pressure 110/73, pulse 120. He has exquisite tenderness in his right costo-vertebral angle. His urine is loaded with WBC and microscopic examination of an unspun, unstained specimen of urine shows many bacteria.

QUESTIONS

1. PROPER MANAGEMENT OF THE PATIENT AT THIS POINT WOULD BE
   - A. withhold all treatment until the culture result is known
   - B. start treatment with ampicillin
   - C. treat symptomatically with pyridium while waiting on the culture result
   - D. plan IVP, voiding cystoureterogram, and cystocopy

An IVP done after the patient responded to treatment shows a dilated right ureter. Cystocopy reveals a block at the right ureterovesical junction. Surgical re-implantation of the ureter was successful. Histopathology of the tissue removed at the site of obstruction is shown in Figure 2.

2. WHAT IS THE ORGANISM?
   - A. Hookworm (*Necator americanus*)
   - B. *Strongyloides*
   - C. *Ascaris*
   - D. *Schistosoma*
   - E. *Taenia*

3. WHICH OF THE FOLLOWING ARE COMPLICATIONS OF SCHISTOSOMIASIS?
   - A. Hematuria
   - B. Portal hypertension
   - C. Bladder cancer
   - D. Epilepsy
   - E. Dysentery

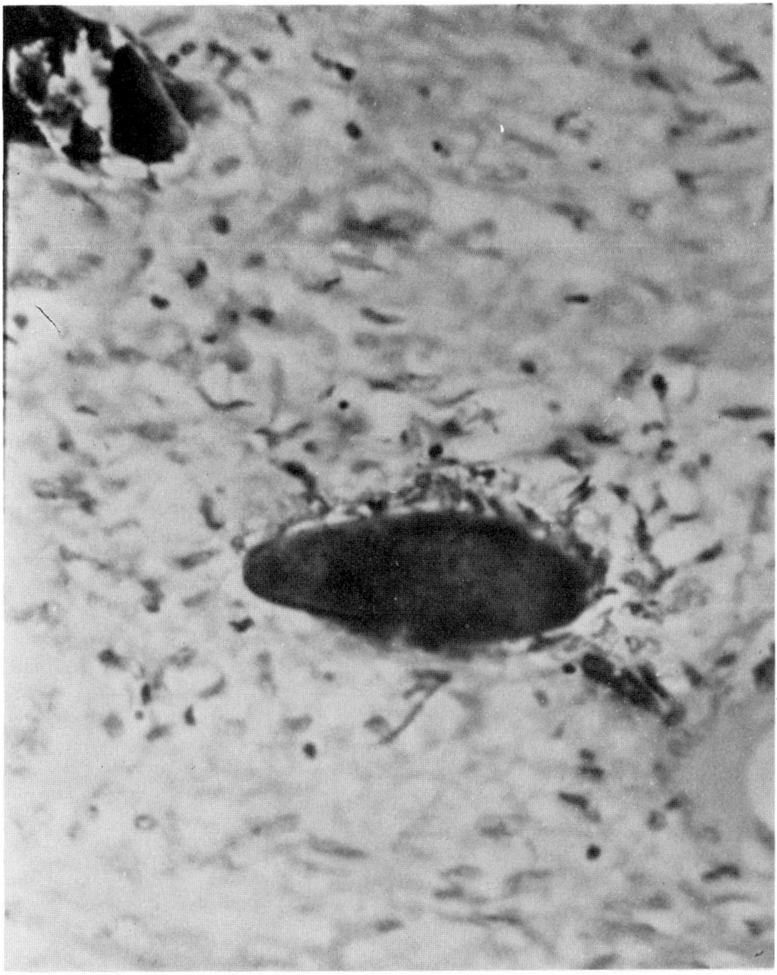

Figure 2

ANSWERS

1. (B, D) The first episode of urinary tract infection in a male of any age warrants a thorough urologic evaluation.

2. (D) *Schistosoma haematobium* is found in most of Africa and normally lives and mates in the veins of the urinary bladder of man with resultant fibrosis and frequent involvement of the ureters and kidneys.

3. (A, B, C, D, E) Hematuria and bladder cancer result from *S. haematobium* infection in the bladder. In Egypt, bladder cancer is the most common cancer in males. *S. mansonii* and *japonicum* produce cirrhosis, dysentery, and CNS involvement.

REFERENCES

1. Mahmond AAF. Current concepts - Schistosomiasis. N Engl J Med 1977; 297:1329.

2. Prata A. Schistosomiasis mansonii. Clin Gastroenterol 1978; 7:49.

3. Warren KS, Mahmoud AAF. Algorithms in the diagnosis and management of exotic diseases. I. Schistosomiasis. J Infect Dis 1975; 131:614.

CASE 58

HISTORY

A 48-year-old diabetic woman is hospitalized because of an ear infection. Three months previously she noted the onset of redness, swelling and drainage from her left ear. The condition has been treated by her local physician with medications unknown to the patient but she has continued to worsen. In the week prior to admission there has been increasing pain and swelling and daily fever.

EXAMINATION

Physical examination reveals an acutely ill woman whose oral temperature is 102°F. There is a considerable amount of drainage from the right ear, and granulation tissue is observed on the floor of the external auditory canal. Gram-negative rods and a few gram-positive cocci in clumps are noted on Gram stained smear of the inflammatory debris.

QUESTIONS

1. INITIAL ANTIMICROBIAL THERAPY SHOULD INCLUDE
   A. topical antimicrobial ointments
   B. parenteral ampicillin
   C. parenteral anti-pseudomonas drugs
   D. parenteral anti-staphylococcal therapy
   E. systemic amphotericin B

Cultures reveal *Pseudomonas aeruginosa*, susceptible to carbenicillin, ticarcillin, gentamicin, tobramycin and amikacin, and resistant to other antimicrobial agents, and coagulase positive *Staphylococcus aureus*, resistant to penicillin G and sensitive to penicillinase resistant penicillins. The patient's fasting blood sugar is 250 mg%.

2. WHICH OF THE FOLLOWING STATEMENTS IS/ARE TRUE?
   A. *Pseudomonas aeruginosa* infection is an unusual cause of chronic otitis externa
   B. The syndrome described in the patient above, "malignant external otitis", is associated with a mortality rate of approximately 50%
   C. Patients with diabetes mellitus have decreased concentrations of circulating immunoglobulins, accounting for an increased susceptibility to infection

D. The most common serious complication of malignant external otitis is cranial nerve palsy
E. Diabetic patients with chronic pseudomonas otitis externa unresponsive to outpatient therapy should probably be hospitalized for intensive treatment

ANSWERS

1. (A, C, D) This clinical syndrome, sometimes called malignant external otitis, is a serious one requiring systemic antimicrobial therapy. Since Pseudomonas aeruginosa is a common pathogen in these circumstances, the attending physician should include antimicrobial therapy directed against it in initial therapy. Anti-staphylococcal therapy should also be included because of the findings on the Gram stain. Topical antibiotic ointments may help and probably won't hurt. Ampicillin and amphotericin B are inappropriate initial choices.

2. (B, D, E) While patients with controlled diabetes mellitus have never unequivocally been shown to have increased susceptibility to infection, most clinicians believe they do. In diabetic ketoacidosis polymorphonuclear leukocyte function is probably abnormal. Several investigators have demonstrated abnormalities of the acute inflammatory response in diabetic patients by use of the Rebuck skin window technique. In addition, defective leukotactic activity of leukocytes from diabetic patients has been demonstrated in vitro as well. Facial nerve palsy is probably the most common complication of malignant external otitis. A recent discussion of this disorder recommends hospitalization in the circumstances outlined above.

REFERENCES

1. Howie VM. Otitis media and externa. In: Mandell GL, Douglas RG Jr, and Bennett JE, eds. Principles and Practices of Infectious Diseases. New York: John Wiley & Sons, 1979; 450-457.

2. Wilson DF, Pulec JL, Linthicum FH Jr. Malignant external otitis. Arch Otolaryng 1971; 93:419.

3. Brayton RG, Stokes PE, Schwartz MS, Louria DB. Effect of alcohol and various diseases on leukocyte mobilization, phagocytosis and intracellular bacterial killing. New Engl J Med 1970; 282:123.

4. Mowat AG, Baum J. Chemotaxis of polymorphonuclear leukocytes from patients with diabetes mellitus. New Engl J Med 1971; 284:621.

5. Zaky DA, Bentley DW, Lowy K, et al. Malignant external otitis: A severe form of otitis in diabetic patients. Am J Med 1976; 61:298.

CASE 59

HISTORY

A 23-year-old black male is hospitalized because of fever. He was in excellent health until one month earlier when he began to experience daily fever to 102°F associated with evening sweats. These symptoms continued to the time of admission.

EXAMINATION

Physical examination reveals a non-ill appearing man with a temperature of 101°F. Otherwise, the physical examination is normal.

LABORATORY DATA

Laboratory evaluation reveals an hematocrit of 33% and a white blood cell count of 9,000 with a normal differential. Uninalysis and chest roentgenogram are normal. The SGOT is 55, alkaline phosphatase 250, bilirubin 2, and calcium 10. Serum protein electrophoresis reveals an albumin of 3 gm% and a gammaglobulin of 2.4 gm% with a diffuse pattern. Chest roentgenogram, liver-spleen scan and gall bladder x-rays are normal. Intermediate strength PPD is negative. Liver biopsy reveals several non-caseating granulomata. Blood cultures are sterile.

QUESTIONS

1. AT THIS POINT, WHICH OF THE FOLLOWING MEASURES IS INDICATED?
   - A. Isoniazid and ethambutol
   - B. Corticosteroids
   - C. Salicylates
   - D. Metronidazole
   - E. None of the above

2. CAUSES OF NON-CASEATING GRANULOMATOUS HEPATITIS INCLUDE WHICH OF THE FOLLOWING?
   - A. Mycobacterium tuberculosis
   - B. Sarcoidosis
   - C. Certain drugs, e.g. sulfonamides
   - D. Berylliosis
   - E. Inflammatory bowel disease
   - F. Lymphoma
   - G. Metastatic carcinoma
   - H. Histoplasmosis
   - I. Q fever
   - J. Tularemia
   - K. Brucellosis

3. WHICH OF THE FOLLOWING STATEMENTS IS/ARE TRUE?

A. The diagnosis of sarcoidosis can be ruled out in a patient who has a normal chest roentgenogram
B. The most sensitive test for pulmonary dysfunction due to sarcoidosis is CO-diffusion capacity of the lung
C. Non-caseating hepatic granulomata secondary to lymphoma occur only when there is infiltration of the liver with lymphoma
D. The presence of non-caseating granulomata in the right supraclavicular lymph node of a patient with a reticular pulmonary infiltrate and right hilar adenopathy establishes the diagnosis of sarcoidosis
E. In disseminated tuberculosis, culture of a percutaneous liver biopsy specimen is more likely than culture of bone marrow to reveal Mycobacterium tuberculosis
F. The finding of a negative intermediate strength PPD in a non-anergic patient with an upper lobe pulmonary infiltrate means that the odds of the patient's having pulmonary tuberculosis are less than 1%

ANSWERS

1. (E) A definitive diagnosis has not been made. A variety of disorders which may cause fever of unknown origin (FUO) also cause non-caseating hepatic granulomata. These include tuberculosis, systemic fungal infections, lymphoma, sarcoidosis, and most forms of systemic immunologic diseases. Further studies, beginning with bone marrow aspiration, biopsy, and culture; gastrointestinal roentgenograms; abdominal CT scan; serologic titers for brucellosis and fungi; immunologic studies such as erythrocyte sedimentation rate and anti-nuclear antibody determination; and pulmonary function studies, looking for depressed DL_{CO} suggestive of sarcoidosis, are indicated in this patient in an attempt to establish a definitive diagnosis. Depending upon the results of the above tests, the physician may wish to obtain further invasive test(s), e.g. arteriograms or biopsies; may begin a "therapeutic trial", e.g. INH for disseminated tuberculosis; may elect to follow the patient without treatment for a period of time; or may have mounted sufficient evidence against an infectious or neoplastic disorder and in favor of sarcoidosis to begin corticosteroids.

It is difficult to establish a defined set of criteria for the diagnostic and therapeutic management of patients with FUO. Therefore, approaches must be tailored to the individual patient and should be guided by the historical and physical findings and the results of screening laboratory tests, especially if there are findings pointing to a specific organ system or region of the body. After a careful, thorough evaluation of such patients, rational decisions regarding whether or not to perform an invasive procedure and, if so, which one(s) can usually be made. However, even in experienced hands, a definitive diagnosis cannot be made in 5-10% of patients with FUO.

2. (A-K) As discussed above.

3. (B,E) The vast majority of, but not all, patients with sarcoidosis have abnormal chest roentgenograms. Non-caseating granulomata may occur at sites distant to the site of primary involvement. Thus, hepatic granulomata may occur in patients with lymphoma that is localized, for example, to the retroperitoneum, and granulomata may develop in regional lymph nodes draining a tissue or organ housing a carcinoma, e. g. a granulomata in a supraclavicular lymph node may be seen in a patient with carcinoma of the lung. Culture of a percutaneous liver biopsy specimen is somewhat more likely to provide a diagnosis of disseminated tuberculosis than is culture of bone marrow, though both specimens are useful. Approximately 20% of patients with pulmonary tuberculosis initially have negative PPD skin tests even though they can react to other skin test antigens. This "selective anergy" usually disappears after a few months of anti-tuberculous therapy.

REFERENCES

1. Guckian JC, Perry JE. Granulomatous hepatitis. An analysis of 63 cases and review of the literature. Ann Intern Med 1966; 65:1081.

2. Simon HB, Wolff SM. Granulomatous hepatitis and prolonged fever of unknown origin: a study of 13 patients. Medicine 1973; 52:1.

3. Israel HL, Goldstein RA. Hepatic granulomatosis and sarcoidosis. Ann Intern Med 1973; 79:669.

4. Mir-Madjlessi SH, Farmer RG, Hawk WA. Granulomatous hepatitis. A review of 50 cases. Am J Gastroenterol 1973; 57:122.

5. Cucin RL, Coleman M, Eckardt JJ, et al. The diagnosis of miliary tuberculosis: Utility of peripheral blood abnormalities, bone marrow and liver needle biopsies. J Chron Dis 1973; 26:355.

6. Kent DC, Schwartz R. Active pulmonary tuberculosis with negative tuberculin skin reactions. Am Rev Resp Dis 1967; 95: 411.

CASE 60

HISTORY

A 23-year-old woman who three months ago moved to the United States from Punjab, India, presents to the hospital complaining of the abrupt onset, two days ago, of a rigor and fever, which lasted about an hour and was followed by a drenching sweat. The day before admission she was afebrile. The morning of admission she again had a rigor and her temperature reached 103°F. She has had similar symptoms on several occasions in the past four years, treated with tablets for 4-5 days.

EXAMINATION

On physical examination the patient was in moderate distress. The temperature was 104°F, the pulse 110, the blood pressure 114/60. There was no rash. The spleen tip was barely palpable.

LABORATORY DATA

The hematocrit was 33%. The WBC count was 5000 with 41% polys and 54% lymphocytes. Urinalysis was normal.

QUESTIONS

1. APPROPRIATE DIAGNOSTIC TESTS WOULD BE
   - A. serology for dengue
   - B. stool for ova and parasites
   - C. blood cultures
   - D. thick and thin smears of peripheral blood
   - E. PPD skin test

2. PLASMODIUM VIVAX WERE SEEN ON BLOOD SMEAR. TREATMENT SHOULD CONSIST OF
   - A. aspirin and observation of benign tertian malaria
   - B. chloroquine alone
   - C. chloroquine and primaquine
   - D. quinine, pyrimethamine, and sulfadiazene

3. A FRIEND IS PLANNING EXTENSIVE TRAVEL IN PANAMA. WHAT TYPE OF MALARIA PROPHYLAXIS SHOULD SHE TAKE?
   - A. Chloroquine weekly
   - B. Quinine daily
   - C. Pyrimethamine-sulfadoxine every other week
   - D. Primaquine weekly
   - E. If pregnant, she can not safely take chloroquine

ANSWERS

1. (C, D)

2. (C) Vivax malaria requires drugs directed at both the erythrocytic and hepatic stage of infection. Chloroquine-resistant malaria is treated with quinine, pyrimethamine, and sulfadiazene.

3. (C) Chloroquine is used for chemoprophylaxis in areas free of resistant falciparum malaria. In those countries of Central and South America where chloroquine resistance occurs, a combination of pyrimethamine-sulfadoxine (Fansidar) may be purchased over-the-counter; it is not available in the United States. Chloroquine is safe during pregnancy.

REFERENCES

1. Chemoprophylaxis of malaria. Morbidity & Mortality Weekly Report 1978; 27:81.

2. Butler T, Warren KS, Mahmoud AAF. Algorithms in the diagnosis and management of exotic disease. XIII. Malaria. J Infect Dis 1976; 133:721.

3. Heineman HS. The clinical syndrome of malaria in the United States. Arch Intern Med 1972; 124:607.

4. Kean BH, Reilly PC Jr. Malaria - the mime: Recent lessons from a group of civilian travellers. Am J Med 1976; 61: 159.

CASE 61

HISTORY

A 45-year-old woman is hospitalized because of fever of one week's duration. She had aortic valve replacement 4 weeks earlier for aortic valve incompetence secondary to rheumatic heart disease. She had received prophylactic therapy with a cephalosporin for 7 days in the peri-operative period. Her post-operative course had been uncomplicated and she had been discharged on the 10th post-operative day on digoxin and coumadin. She was well until one week prior to admission when she noted malaise and afternoon fever to 102°F. These symptoms persisted until the time of admission.

EXAMINATION

Physical examination reveals a mildly ill appearing woman with a temperature of 102°F. Cardiovascular examination is normal; the prosthetic valve sounds are normal. The liver is palpable two finger breadths below the right costal margin and is tender. The remainder of the physical examination is normal.

LABORATORY DATA

The white blood cell count is 15,000 with 45% polymorphonuclear leukocytes and 50% lymphocytes, half of which are atypical. SGOT is 200; blood cultures are drawn.

QUESTIONS

1. THE MOST LIKELY DIAGNOSIS IS
   - A. infectious endocarditis
   - B. toxoplasmosis
   - C. cytomegalovirus infection
   - D. infectious mononucleosis
   - E. fever and hepatitis secondary to coumadin
   - F. hepatitis due to either hepatitis B or non-A, non-B hepatitis virus

2. WHICH OF THE FOLLOWING DISORDERS MAY BE ACQUIRED FROM BLOOD TRANSFUSIONS?
   - A. Cytomegalovirus infection
   - B. Syphilis
   - C. Malaria
   - D. Viral hepatitis
   - E. Tuberculosis
   - F. Chagas' disease (South American trypanosomiasis)

3. WHICH OF THE FOLLOWING STATEMENTS IS/ARE TRUE?

A. Only women who acquire cytomegalovirus infection during or immediately preceding pregnancy are at risk of transmitting cytomegalovirus infection to their fetuses
B. Only women who acquire rubella infection during or immediately preceding pregnancy are at risk of transmitting rubella to their fetuses
C. Only women who acquire *Toxoplasma gondii* infection during or immediately preceding pregnancy are at risk of transmitting toxoplasmosis to their fetuses
D. Only women who acquire syphilis during or immediately preceding pregnancy are at risk of transmitting syphilis to their fetuses
E. The first trimester is the chief time during which *Treponema pallidum* is transmitted from mother to fetus

ANSWERS

1. (C) While prosthetic valve endocarditis is a major concern, the absence of cardiac findings and of peripheral signs of endocarditis and the presence of atypical lymphocytes argue strongly against that diagnosis. Her illness is consistent with the mononucleosis syndrome, which may be caused by Ebstein-Barr virus, cytomegalovirus, *Toxoplasma gondii*, hepatitis viruses, and less commonly by adenovirus, herpes simplex, and brucellae. The most likely cause of this patient's illness is cytomegalovirus, acquired from blood used during bypass surgery.

2. (A, B, C, D, F)

3. (B, C) While *Toxoplasma gondii* and rubella virus circulate only in association with the primary infection, cytomegalovirus and even *T. pallidum* can circulate months later and can infect a fetus at times remote from the primary infection of the mother. Only after about four months of gestation will the placenta permit entry of *T. pallidum*; therefore, the fetus is usually safe until the second trimester.

REFERENCES

1. Lang DJ, Hanshaw JB. Cytomegalovirus infection and the post-perfusion syndrome. Recognition of primary infections in four patients. New Engl J Med 1969; 280:1145.

2. Foster KM, Jack I. A prospective study of the role of cytomegalovirus in post-transfusion mononucleosis. New Engl J Med 1969; 280:1311.

3. Stagno S, Reynolds DW, Huang E-S, et al. Congenital cytomegalovirus infection. Occurrence in an immune population. New Engl J Med 1977; 296:1254.

4. Naeye RL, Blanc W. Pathogenesis of congenital rubella. J Am Med Assn 1965; 194:1277.

5. Desmonts G, Couvreur J. Congenital toxoplasmosis: A prospective study of 378 pregnancies. New Engl J Med 1974; 290:1110.

6. Al-Salihi FL, Curran JP, Shetein OA. Occurrence of fetal syphilis after a nonreactive early gestational serologic test. J Pediatr 1971; 78:121.

CASE 62

HISTORY

A fourteen-month-old boy was referred from another hospital for infected ventriculo-peritoneal shunt. The baby was born prematurely and had meningomyelocele and hydrocephalus. He underwent his first shunt when he was seven weeks old. One week prior to transfer he was admitted to an outside hospital because of fever. Needle aspiration of the shunt revealed cloudy fluid which grew Staphylococcus epidermidis resistant to methicillin and nafcillin but susceptible to cephalothin.

QUESTIONS

1. ALL OF THE FOLLOWING STATEMENTS REGARDING BACTERIAL INFECTION COMPLICATING SHUNTS USED TO TREAT HYDROCEPHALUS ARE TRUE EXCEPT
   - A. cure of bacterial ventriculitis is unusual unless the shunt is removed
   - B. infection of a ventriculo-peritoneal shunt may cause localized or diffuse peritonitis
   - C. E. coli is the most common cause of ventriculo-atrial shunt infection
   - D. cephalosporins administered parenterally are reasonable alternatives for treatment of staphylococcal shunt infection and ventriculitis when the staphylococcus is susceptible to semi-synthetic penicillinase-resistant penicillins and the patient has a history of skin rash following penicillin
   - E. chronic shunt infection may be associated with immune complex disease

2. WHICH OF THE FOLLOWING STATEMENTS REGARDING STAPHYLOCOCCUS EPIDERMIDIS IS/ARE TRUE?
   - A. This bacterial species comprises a significant portion of the normal flora of the skin
   - B. It is more commonly resistant to penicillinase-resistant semi-synthetic penicillins than is Staphylococcus aureus
   - C. It is less virulent than Staphylococcus aureus
   - D. It is the most common contaminant of blood cultures
   - E. It is the most common cause of prosthetic heart valve infection

3. WHICH OF THE FOLLOWING STATEMENTS REGARDING ANTIMICROBIAL PHARMACOLOGY IS/ARE TRUE?
   - A. Neither clindamycin nor cephalothin achieve predictable levels in cerebrospinal fluid whether or not there is meningeal inflammation

B. Cephaloridine may be utilized intraventricularly/intrathecally for therapy of staphylococcal meningitis
C. When vancomycin is administered parenterally sufficient levels appear in the cerebrospinal fluid to kill most strains of Staphylococcus aureus
D. Intrathecal administration of aminoglycosides (e.g. gentamicin) via the lumbar sac is adequate treatment for ventriculitis caused by susceptible aerobic gram-negative bacilli
E. Amphotericin B must be administered intrathecally or intraventricularly for effective therapy of cryptococcal meningitis

ANSWERS

1. (A, B, E) As a rule bacterial infections involving foreign bodies are difficult to erradicate unless the foreign body is removed. This is true in the case of infected ventriculo-atrial shunts. When a ventriculo-peritoneal shunt is in place ventriculitis may cause inoculation of the peritoneal cavity by potentially pathogenic microorganisms which may then produce localized or generalized peritonitis. Staphylococcus epidermidis is the most common etiologic microorganism recovered from the cerebrospinal fluid of patients with infected ventriculo-atrial shunts. It is responsible for 60-90% of such infections. Approximately one half of these patients become ill in the first two months after shunt placement but others may become sick months to years later. Parenteral administration of cephalosporin drugs does not predictably give CSF levels which are adequate for therapy of ventriculitis or meningitis (see below). There have been a number of reports of immune complex disease following chronic shunt infections. The pathogenesis is presumably similar to that which occurs in patients with infective endocarditis.

2. (A, B, C, D, E) Staphylococcus epidermidis is the most common aerobic microorganism which can be recovered from the skin of normal humans and it is a common contaminant of blood cultures. By most criteria Staphylococcus epidermidis is less virulent than Staphylococcus aureus. Although less virulent, Staphylococcus epidermidis is paradoxically more resistant than Staphylococcus aureus to the penicillinase-resistant semi-synthetic penicillins such as nafcillin and methicillin. Whereas fewer than 5% of Staphylococcus aureus strains in the United States are resistant to methicillin, as many as 50% of strains of Staphylococcus epidermidis from the same laboratories are resistant to that drug. In addition, while strains of Staphylococcus aureus which are resistant to methicillin are almost always

resistant to the cephalosporins, this is not always the case with Staphylococcus epidermidis. Staphylococcus epidermidis is responsible for approximately 25% of episodes of prosthetic valve endocarditis, representing a greater proportion than any other bacteria.

3. (A, B) Clindamycin and the cephalosporins are unacceptable antimicrobial agents for therapy of central nervous system disease because of their poor penetration into the subarachnoid space. In contrast, cephalosporins may be utilized for intraventricular or intrathecal therapy of staphylococcal meningitis. In this circumstance cephaloradine is frequently employed. It is important to emphasize that cephaloradine is not recommended for parenteral therapy in any circumstance because of serious nephrotoxicity which has resulted from its use. In addition there is some evidence that the combination of cephalosporins and aminoglycosides is more nephrotoxic than expected from individual toxicities. Vancomycin levels in cerebrospinal fluid are marginal even in the circumstance of inflamed meninges when the drug is administered parenterally. Likewise the aminoglycoside agents such as gentamicin, tobramycin, kanamycin and streptomycin do not reliably give adequate cerebrospinal fluid levels when administered parenterally and are not appropriate therapy by that route for bacterial meningitis. Parenteral amphotericin B in combination with 5 flurocytosine is appropriate therapy for most patients with cryptococcal meningitis, and intraventricular or intrathecal therapy is not usually required for this disorder. In contrast, patients with coccidioidal meningitis should receive both parenteral and intrathecal/intraventricular/intracisternal therapy.

REFERENCES

1. Mandell GL. Cephalosporins. In: Mandell GL, Douglas RG Jr, and Bennett JE, eds. Principles and Practices of Infectious Diseases. New York: John Wiley & Sons, 1979; 238-47.

2. Barza M. The nephrotoxicity of cephalosporins: An overview. J Infect Dis 1978; 137:S60.

3. Wade JC, Petty BG, Conrad G, et al. Cephalothin plus an aminoglyside is more nephrotoxic than methicillin plus an aminoglycoside. Lancet 1978; 604.

4. Fekety R. Vancomycin. In: Mandell GL, Douglas RG Jr. and Bennett JE, eds. Principles and Practices of Infectious Diseases. New York: John Wiley & Sons, 1979; 304-07.

5. Lindholm DD, Murray JS. Persistence of vancomycin in the blood during renal failure and its treatment by hemodialysis. N Engl J Med 1966; 274:1047.

6. Hawley HB, Gump DW. Vancomycin therapy of bacterial meningitis. Am J Dis Child 1973; 126:261.

7. Eykyn S, Philip I, Evans J. Vancomycin for staphylococcal shunt infections in patients on regular hemodialysis. Brit Med J 1970; 3:80.

8. Nielsen HE, Hansen HE, Korsager B, et al. Renal excretion of vancomycin in kidney disease. Acta Med Scand 1975; 197:261.

9. Korzeniowski OM, Hook EW. Aminocyclitols: Aminoglycosides and spectinomycin. In: Mandell GL, Douglas RG Jr, and Bennett JE, eds. Principles and Practices of Infectious Diseases. New York: John Wiley & Sons, 1979; 249-72.

10. Steigbigel NH. Erythromycin, lincomycin, and clindamycin. In: Mandell GL, Douglas RG Jr, and Bennett JE, eds. Principles and Practices of Infectious Diseases. New York: John Wiley & Sons, 1979; 290-300.

11. Panzer JD, Brown DC, Epstein WL, et al. Clindamycin levels in various body tissues and fluids. J Clin Pharm 1972; 12:259.

12. Shurtleff DB, Foltz, EL, Weeks, RD, Lueser, J. Therapy of staphylococcus epidermidis: infections associated with associated with cerebrospinal fluid shunts. Pediatrics 1974; 53: 55.

13. Rames L, Wise B, Goodman JR, Piel CF. Renal disease with Staphylococcus albus bacteremia: A complication in ventriculo-atrial shunts. J Am Med Assn 1970; 212:1671.

14. Archer GL. Antimicrobial susceptibility and selection of resistance among Staphylococcus epidermidis isolates recovered from patients with infections of indwelling foreign devices. Antimicrob Agents Chemother 1978; 14:353.

15. Lerner PI. Penetration of cephalothin and lincomycin into the cerebrospinal fluid. Am J Med Sci 1969; 257:125.

16. Silverblatt F. Nephrotoxicity due to cephaloradine: A light- and electron-microscopic study in rabbits. J Inf Dis 1970; 122:33.

17. Pulverer G, Damen G, Neugebauer M. Antibiotic resistance of Staphylococcus albus. Med Microbiol Immunol 1972; 158:32.

18. Shoenbaum SC, Gardner P, Shillito J. Infections of cerebrospinal fluid shunts: Epidemiology, clinical manifestations and therapy. J Inf Dis 1975; 131: 543.

CASE 63

HISTORY

A 60-year-old woman with long standing diabetes mellitus is hospitalized with a foot ulcer which was first noticed 6 weeks earlier. Despite therapy with elevation and soaks, it progressed such that it is now 7 cm in diameter with a surrounding 10 cm zone of cellulitis.

EXAMINATION

All toes of the foot appear nonviable and there is a tender cord in the calf. Her temperature is 101°F. A putrid odor fills her room.

LABORATORY DATA

Gram's stain of purulent drainage from the base of the ulcer reveals gram-positive cocci in chains, thin filamentous gram-negative bacilli, and broader gram-negative bacilli.

QUESTIONS

1. WHICH OF THE FOLLOWING IS/ARE REASONABLE INITIAL ANTIMICROBIAL REGIMEN(S)?
   - A. A cephalosporin and gentamicin
   - B. A cephalosporin and chloramphenicol
   - C. Chloramphenicol and gentamicin
   - D. Clindamycin
   - E. Clindamycin and gentamicin
   - F. Nafcillin and gentamicin

Blood cultures are obtained, the ulcer is debrided, and therapy is begun with appropriate antimicrobial agents and heparin. On the third day she remains febrile and develops dyspnea, cough productive of bloody sputum, hypoxemia, and an infiltrate in the lateral basal segment of the right lower lobe.

2. APPROPRIATE THERAPY INCLUDES
   - A. immediate amputation of the involved leg above the area of infection and phlebitis
   - B. vena cava interruption
   - C. stopping heparin
   - D. administration of oxygen
   - E. administration of corticosteroids
   - F. administration of digoxin

3. WHICH OF THE FOLLOWING STATEMENTS IS/ARE TURE?

A. When the decision to employ venous interruption is made in order to control septic pulmonary emboli from pelvic infection in a woman, one should ligate the ovarian veins as well as the inferior vena cava
B. Bacteroides bacteremia is associated with jaundice because it elaborates a toxin which causes massive hemolysis
C. Bacteroides infections frequently cause thrombophlebitis
D. The most common antecedent site of infection resulting in bacteroides bacteremia is a cutaneous ulcer
E. Bacteroides urinary tract infections are associated with alkaline urine because bacteroides split urea to ammonia

ANSWERS

1. (B, C, E) The findings of a putrid odor and mixed flora on Gram's stain strongly suggest that infection is caused by a combination of aerobic and anaerobic bacteria. Therefore, any antimicrobial regimen that provides broad anaerobic coverage and coverage for most aerobic gram-negative bacilli is appropriate initial therapy. The choices indicated fit these criteria.

2. (A, B, C, D) The patient almost certainly has had a pulmonary embolus with infarction. Since this life threatening event occurred while she was receiving appropriate antimicrobial therapy and anticoagulation, removal of the source of the embolus and vena cava interruption are indicated. Heparin should be discontinued only during the peri-operative period.

3. (A, C) Since the ovarian veins often enter the vena cava above the level at which vena cava ligation is accomplished, they should be ligated individually. Bacteroides is a frequent cause of infectious thrombophlebitis. Bacteroides bacteremia is commonly associated with jaundice, but jaundice is due to metastatic bacteroides infection in the liver, not to hemolysis. The most common site of anaerobic infection is the peritoneal cavity. Proteus species, not bacteroides, are urea splitters. Bacteroides are an extremely uncommon cause of urinary tract infection.

REFERENCES

1. Louie TJ, Bartlett JG, Tally FP, Gorbach SL. Aerobic and anaerobic bacteria in diabetic foot ulcers. Ann Intern Med 1976; 85:461.

2. Ledger WJ. The surgical care of severe infections in obstetric and gynecologic patients. Surg Gynec Obstet 1973; 132: 753.

3. Bosio BB, Taylore ES. Bacteroides and puerperal infection. Obstet Gynecol 1973; 42:271.

4. Rotheram EB, Schick SF. Nonclostridial anaerobic bacteremia in septic abortion. Am J Med 1969; 46:80.

5. Nobels FR Jr. Bacteroides infections. Ann Surg 1973; 177:601.

6. Chow AW, Guze LB. Bacteroidaceae bacteremia - clinical experience with 112 patients. Medicine 1974; 53:93.

CASE 64

HISTORY

A 23-year-old woman presents to her private physician because of back pain, fever and dysuria of three days' duration. One year previously, while on her honeymoon, she had an episode of "cystitis". She received a short course of sulfonamides and became asymptomatic within a few days. Six months later she had a similar episode and again responded to antimicrobial treatment. Her present episode began three days ago when she again noted dysuria, urgency and blood-tinged urine. The following day she noted fever and bilateral flank pain.

EXAMINATION

Physical examination at the present time reveals a temperature of 102°F, bilateral flank tenderness and supra-pubic tenderness. Urinalysis reveals many white blood cells and white blood cell casts; Gram's stain of the uncentrifuged urine reveals numerous gram-negative rods per high power field.

QUESTIONS

1. WHICH OF THE FOLLOWING IS/ARE APPROPRIATE?
   A. Urine culture and colony count
   B. Immediate initiation of antimicrobial therapy to be continued for 10 days
   C. Intravenous pyelogram
   D. Cystoscopic examination
   E. Evaluation of renal function

Intravenous pyelogram and cystoscopic examination are performed and there is no evidence of anatomic abnormality in the urinary tract. E. coli in a titer of 100,000 colonies per ml is recovered from the urine and treatment is initiated with sulfonamide. Within three days the patient becomes asymptomatic, and after two weeks the ampicillin is discontinued. Two weeks after cessation of therapy a urine culture and colony count reveals 100,000 colonies of Proteus mirabilis, sensitive to ampicillin and gentamicin but resistant to sulfonamides.

2. APPROPRIATE MANAGEMENT AT THIS TIME WOULD BE
   A. since the patient is asymptomatic, she should be followed without specific therapy
   B. she should be admitted to the hospital and treated with parenteral gentamicin

C. she should receive a 10-14 day course of ampicillin
D. she should be placed on trimethoprim-sulfamethoxazole for 6 months

3. WHICH OF THE FOLLOWING IS/ARE TRUE?
A. Asymptomatic bacteriuria in pregnancy is associated with premature delivery
B. The prevalence of bacteriuria of pregnancy declines with age and parity
C. One out of five women who have asymptomatic bacteriuria early in pregnancy will develop acute symptomatic peylonephritis later in pregnancy
D. An intravenous pyelogram may reveal dilated ureters in normal post-partum women up to six weeks after delivery
E. In most cases bacteriuria cannot be eradicated in a patient with urinary tract obstruction until the obstruction is relieved

ANSWERS

1. (A, B, C, D, E) Many aspects of the pathogenesis, management and implications of recurrent urinary tract infection are unclear. A patient such as this one should have a 'work up' to exclude correctable anatomic abnormalities. Urologic consultation may be required for such a 'work up'. If no correctable lesions are found, a short course (i. e. 10 days - 2 weeks) of appropriate antimicrobial therapy would be reasonable. Some authors recommend a single-dose course of therapy for bacteriuria with further work up and treatment of the 30% who fail to respond to this brief regimen.

2. (C) If the infecting organism is resistant to the commonly used oral preparations, then the patient should be hospitalized for parenteral therapy. If this second two-week course of treatment fails to eradicate bacteriuria, long-term suppressive therapy must be considered. In this patient the pattern of recurrent bacteriuria with different organisms represents <u>reinfection</u> rather than <u>relapse</u>.

3. (A, C, D, E) Because of the frequent development of pyelonephritis in pregnant women with asymptomatic bacteriuria, a goal of prenatal care is to maintain a sterile urine throughout pregnancy.

REFERENCES

1. Andriole VT. Urinary tract infection in pregnancy. Urol Clin N Am 1975; 2:485.

2. Little PJ. The incidence of urinary infection in 5000 women. Lancet 1966; 2:925.

3. Fang LST, Tolkoff NE, Rubin RH. Efficacy of single-dose and conventional amoxicillin therapy in urinary-tract infection localized by the antibody-coated bacteria technic. New Engl J Med 1978; 298:413.

4. Turck M, Anderson KN, Petersdorf RG. Relapse and reinfection in chronic bacteriuria. New Engl J Med 1966; 275:70.

5. Santoro J, Kaye D. Recurrent urinary tract infections. Pathogenesis and management. Med Clin N Am 1978; 62:1005.

6. Zinner SH, Kass EH. Long-term (10-14 yrs) follow-up of bacteriuria of pregnancy. New Engl J Med 1971; 285:820.

CASE 65

HISTORY

A 16-year-old, previously healthy woman is hospitalized because of abdominal pain of 18 hours' duration. Physical examination and laboratory findings are consistent with the diagnosis of appendicitis and laparotomy via a McBurney's incision is performed. At laparotomy the appendix appears normal but the para-cecal lymph nodes are inflamed. One of the lymph nodes is excised and sent for pathologic examination and culture.

QUESTIONS

1. WHICH OF THE FOLLOWING INFECTIOUS AGENTS IS THE MOST LIKELY CAUSE OF THE PATIENT'S ILLNESS?
   - A. *Mycobacterium tuberculosis*
   - B. A non-tuberculous mycobacterium
   - C. *Yersinia pseudotuberculosis*
   - D. *Vibrio parahemolyticus*
   - E. *Escherichia coli*
   - F. *Entameba histolytica*

The patient has an uneventful intra-operative course and is returned to her room. No antibiotic is administered. Twelve hours post-operatively, the patient has a chill and fever to 106° F. On physical examination, the patient appears acutely ill, is tachypneic and has a tachycardia of 120 beats/min. The surgical wound and surrounding area are erythematous and exquisitely tender.

2. THE MOST LIKELY CAUSE OF THE PATIENT'S CURRENT ILLNESS IS
   - A. group A streptococcus
   - B. a reaction to the anesthetic
   - C. *Enterobacter agglomerans* bacteremia originating from the contents of the intravenous fluid bottle
   - D. *Staphylococcus aureus*
   - E. malignant hyperthermia
   - F. dissemination of one of the microorganisms in question 1 above

3. WHICH OF THE FOLLOWING STATEMENTS IS/ARE TRUE?
   - A. The above patient should be placed on contact isolation
   - B. Adenovirus is a rare cause of intussusception and of mesenteric adenitis mimicking acute appendicitis in children

C. Injection of saline into the leading edge of the area of erythema and aspiration of fluid from the subcutaneous tissues may yield material appropriate for Gram's stain and culture of the area of cellulitis
D. The genetic defect in malignant hyperthermia appears to result in an abnormality of muscle cell metabolism
E. Streptococcal cellulitis is readily distinguished clinically from staphylococcal cellulitis; therefore, penicillin G can be employed as initial therapy for cellulitis which is felt to be streptococcal on clinical grounds

ANSWERS

1. (C) The patient has mesenteric adenitis. While *Mycobacterium tuberculosis* can cause cecal and para-cecal disease, the acute onset of this patient's illness suggests that her disease is caused by either *Yersinia pseudotuberculosis*, *Yersinia enterocolitica*, or adenovirus.

2. (A) The patient almost certainly has bacterial wound infection and cellulitis. While nearly any bacterium may be responsible, the development of illness of this magnitude in such a short time strongly suggests group A streptococcal disease.

3. (A, B, C, D) Hospitalized patients with wound infection due to any bacterium should be placed on contact isolation; this is especially true if the causative agent is group A streptococcus or *Staphylococcus aureus*, for spread of infection to other patients by health care personnel is a frequent cause of nosocomial infection. Current evidence suggests that patients who develop malignant hyperthermia after administration of anesthetic agents have an as yet not completely defined disorder of muscle metabolism. One may predict from physical examination with perhaps 70% accuracy that cellulitis in a given patient is due to group A streptococcus and not to *Staphylococcus aureus* or vice versa. However, we have been fooled sufficiently often that we always treat initially with an antimicrobial agent effective against both. After results of culture and susceptibility are known, treatment can be modified appropriately.

REFERENCES

1. Weber J, Finlayson NB, Mark JBD. Mesenteric lymphadenitis and terminal ileitis due to *Yersina pseudotuberculosis*. New Engl J Med 1970; 283:172.

2. Knapp W. Mesenteric adenitis due to *Pasteurella pseudotuberculosis* in young people. New Engl J Med 1958; 259:776.

3. Henshall TC. Pasteurella pseudotuberculosis mesenteric adenitis. New Zeal Med J 1963; 62:462.

4. Duma RJ, Weinberg AN, Medrek TF, Kunz LJ. Streptococcal infections. A bacteriologic and clinical study of streptococcal bacteremia. Medicine 1969; 48:87.

5. Maki DG, Rhame FS, Mackel DC, Bennett JV. Nationwide epidemic of septicemia caused by contaminated intravenous products. I. Epidemiologic and clinical features. Am J Med 1976; 60:471.

6. Moulds RGW. Biochemical basis of malignant hyperthermia. Brit Med J 1974; 2:241.

7. Clarke EJ Jr, Philips IA, Alexander ER. Adenovirus in intussusception in children in Taiwan. J Am Med Assn 1969; 208:1671.

CASE 66

HISTORY

This 23-year-old white female was transferred to the University of Alabama Hospital for fever and headache. She had been well until 3 months previously when she noted the onset of throbbing bitemporal headaches associated with low grade fever. She was treated for "sinusitis" with antibiotics and pain medications. Two months prior to admission the headaches recurred and this time were associated with nausea, vomiting and fever. Because the headaches persisted she was admitted to an outside hospital approximately two weeks prior to transfer. The patient denied prior sinusitus, head trauma or exposure to patients with tuberculosis.

EXAMINATION

On physical examination she was hypertensive and febrile. There was moderate nuchal rigidity and mild obtundation, otherwise the general physical examination and neurologic exam were unremarkable.

LABORATORY DATA

Admission laboratory work revealed a white count of 4700, and an elevated erythrocyte sedimentation rate. Lumbar puncture results are illustrated in Table 1. Because of a weakly positive antinuclear antibody test the patient was begun on corticosteroids and improved transiently during the first four days of therapy but subsequently began complaining again of severe headaches. A second lumbar puncture was done (7/23) because of continued headache, fever, nausea and vomiting and she was transferred to University Hospital. One day prior to transfer she complained of diplopia.

Here the physical examination was unchanged, laboratory work was also similar to that determined at the outside hospital. A third lumbar puncture was done (7/30) and the results are also shown in Table 1.

TABLE 1

Date	Pressure	Cell Count Polys/lymphs	Glucose	Protein
7/17		5/70	45	53
7/23	220	10/100	19	174
7/30	200	90/50	20	250
8/23		10/90	44	284

QUESTIONS

1. ADDITIONAL DIAGNOSTIC MANEUVERS SHOULD INCLUDE
   A. EEG
   B. CT scan
   C. cytospin or cytologic examination of cerebrospinal fluid for determination of cellular morphology
   D. pneumoencephalogram
   E. IPPD skin-test

The intermediate strength PPD was positive.

2. WHICH OF THE FOLLOWING THERAPEUTIC PLANS IS NOW APPROPRIATE?
   A. Initiation of antituberculous therapy
   B. Initiation of anti-fungal therapy with amphotericin B and 5 flurocytosine
   C. Reinitiation of corticosteroid treatment
   D. Broad spectrum antibacterial therapy, e.g. penicillin and chloramphenicol
   E. Anti-viral therapy, i.e. adenine arabanoside (ara A)

Antituberculous therapy was begun and the lumbar puncture was repeated on several occasions. Approximately 3 weeks after being admitted to University Hospital the laboratory from the outside hospital called to report that M. tuberculosis was growing from the initial spinal fluid culture.

3. WHICH OF THE FOLLOWING STATEMENTS IS/ARE TRUE?
   A. Corticosteroids play an important role in the therapy of tuberculous meningitis
   B. Persistent headache, high cerebrospinal fluid pressure and ventricular dilatation demonstrated by CT scan would suggest communicating hydrocephalus. This complication may require ventriculoatrial shunt.

C. Untreated tuberculous meningitis is invariably fatal
D. Acid fast bacilli are usually not seen in initial specimens of cerebrospinal fluid in tuberculous meningitis

ANSWERS

1. (A, B, C, E) Even though expensive, the CT scan is such a valuable tool for determining the presence of focal neurologic disease that it is probably worthwhile obtaining such a study in most patients with undiagnosed central nervous system disease and focal signs. The presence of diplopia in this patient probably warrants the CT scan. In addition an EEG is useful in patients with neurologic disorders to quantify the degree and pattern of cortical electrical disorganization. Cytospin or cytological examination of cells in cerebrospinal fluid is an important adjunctive diagnostic maneuver for patients with chronic or subacute meningitis, especially in the presence of a depressed glucose concentration. This may be combined with a search for B and T cell markers when malignant lymphoma is suspected. The CT scan has abrogated many of the indications for pneumoencephalography and that test is rarely indicated today. An intermediate strength tuberculin skin test would be crucial in this patient even though she has received corticosteroids in the past. If the test were positive it would be very useful for planning therapy. Arteriograms are not appropriate at this time. If a mass lesion were noted on a CT scan they might be more reasonable.

2. (A) Antituberculous therapy should be administered to almost any patient with lymphocytic meningitis, associated with a depressed cerebrospinal fluid glucose and a positive intermediate strength PPD unless the disorder is known to be due to some other non-tuberculous cause. On the other hand, empiric anti-fungal therapy with amphotericin B is generally not indicated until a fungal etiology is "proven" by demonstration of the agent or its antigen in spinal fluid. Corticosteroid therapy should rarely be given in undiagnosed lymphocytic meningitis since it may mask the manifestations of disseminated fungal or tuberculous disease. Antibacterial therapy may be used when brain abscess is suspected; however, in most other disorders associated with chronic lymphocytic meningitis it is not appropriate nor is antiviral therapy.

3. (B, D) A controlled study of corticosteroids in tuberculous meningitis demonstrated no improvement in overall outcome although short term morbidity from cerebral edema was ameliorated somewhat. When headache, high cerebrospinal fluid pressure and dilated ventricles on CT scan suggest communicating

hydrocephalus corticosteroids may be tried. If they are not helpful then neurosurgical consultation should be obtained. See the report by Emond regarding untreated tuberculous meningitis. Approximately two thirds of initial CSF samples from patients with tuberculous meningitis have no demonstrable acid fast organism.

REFERENCES

1. Kennedy DH, Fallon RJ. Tuberculous meningitis. J Am Med Assn 1979; 241:264.

2. Kocen RS, Parsons M. Neurological complications of tuberculosis: Some unusual manifestations. Quart J Med 1970; 29:17.

3. O'Toole RD, Thornton GF, Mukherjee MK, Nath RL. Dexamethasone in tuberculous meningitis: relationship of cerebrospinal fluid effects to therapeutic efficacy. Ann Intern Med 1969; 70:39.

4. Emond RTD. Tuberculosis as a cause of transient aseptic meningitis. Lancet 1973; 2:234.

5. Smith HV. Tuberculous meningitis. Int J Neurology 1964; 4:134.

CASE 67

HISTORY

A 58-year-old man is referred from another hospital because of bacteremia. He had been evaluated six weeks earlier for weight loss, heat intolerance, tachycardia, exophthalmos and thyromegaly. Grave's disease was documented by appropriate studies and he was begun on propylthiouracil with improvement in his symptoms of hypermetabolism and reduction of the serum thyroxin level to normal. Five days prior to admission, he abraded the skin of the left hand at work. Three days prior to admission, he developed fever, erythema, and tenderness of the abrasion site and signs of cellulitis of the dorsum of the hand. He was hospitalized the next day. Gram's stain of the material from the area of cellulitis revealed gram-positive cocci in clusters. Blood cultures were obtained and treatment was begun with nafcillin. The day before transfer, wound and blood cultures grew Staphylococcus aureus.

EXAMINATION

Physical examination at the time of transfer reveals a moderately ill appearing man with a temperature of 103°F. A healing abrasion site of the dorsum of the left third finger is noted. The entire dorsum of the left hand is erythematous and tender. There are erythematous streaks ascending the forearm and the arm. Tender left axillary and epitrochlear adenopathy are present. The remainder of the physical examination is unremarkable.

LABORATORY DATA

The white blood cell count reveals 1500 cells with only 3% polymorphonuclear leukocytes. The remainder are lymphocytes and monocytes. The hematocrit is 40%; platelet count is 250,000.

QUESTIONS

1. THE MOST LIKELY CAUSE OF NEUTROPENIA IN THIS PATIENT IS
   - A. pre-leukemic acute leukemia
   - B. propylthiouracil-induced agranulocytosis
   - C. thyrotoxicosis-induced agranulocytosis
   - D. drug-induced systemic lupus erythematosus
   - E. idiopathic auto-immune neutropenia
   - F. chronic myelogenous leukemia

Propylthiouracil is stopped and treatment with nafcillin continued; the patient becomes afebrile by the third hospital day. At that time, the areas of cellulitis, lymphangitis and lymphadenitis are improved. On the 5th hospital day, the patient has a frank chill and temperature spike to 105°F. Physical examination is unchanged except that he appears more ill. The white blood cell count is the same as on admission. Urinalysis and renal function are normal.

2. AFTER OBTAINING BLOOD CULTURES YOU WOULD
   A. stop nafcillin; begin vancomycin
   B. continue nafcillin
   C. continue nafcillin and add gentamicin
   D. continue nafcillin and add gentamicin and carbenicillin
   E. continue nafcillin; prepare for emergency thyroidectomy for management of thyroid storm

3. WHICH OF THE FOLLOWING STATEMENTS IS/ARE TRUE?
   A. A hemogram obtained on the 12th hospital day revealing a white blood cell count of 4500 with 12% neutrophils, 15% bands, 7% metamyelocytes, 6% myelocytes, 3% blasts and the remainder lymphocytes and monocytes would substantiate the diagnosis of chronic myelogenous leukemia in the patient presented
   B. Carbenicillin and gentamicin are clearly synergistic in vivo in neutropenic patients who have pseudomonas bacteremia
   C. Carbenicillin and gentamicin may be administered in the same intravenous bottle
   D. Oral carbenicillin may be used to treat uncomplicated urinary tract infection caused by susceptible bacteria
   E. High dose, intravenous carbenicillin, employed alone, is appropriate antimicrobial therapy for a patient with pneumonia and bacteremia caused by a carbenicillin-susceptible _Pseudomonas aeruginosa_

ANSWERS

1. (B)

2. (D) It is likely that nafcillin is controlling the patient's staphylococcal disease and that the current problem is not due to staphylococcus. The possible causes of the current problem are a nosocomial superinfection or a reaction to nafcillin. While the latter is possible, there is nothing specific to suggest drug reaction, and nosocomial infection with a gram-negative bacillus seems most likely. We would therefore continue

nafcillin and add gentamicin and carbenicillin. In fact, blood cultures obtained at this time subsequently grew Klebsiella pneumoniae.

3. (B, D) Patients whose bone marrow is recovering from a severe insult usually develop leukocytosis with a marked left shift, occasionally including the transient appearance of a few blast forms. The combination of carbenicillin and gentamicin is clearly more efficacious than gentamicin alone in granulocytopenic patients with pseudomonas bacteremia. When mixed in the same intravenous bottle, carbenicillin inactivates gentamicin. Many isolates of Pseudomonas aeruginosa become rapidly resistant to carbenicillin when that agent is employed alone; therefore, an aminoglycoside should be added.

REFERENCES

1. Young LS, Martin WJ, Meyer RD, et al. Gram-negative rod bacteremia: Microbiologic, immunologic, and therapeutic considerations. Ann Intern Med 1977; 86:456.

2. Finland M, Barnes MW. Bacteremic superinfections of patients with bacteremia: Occurrence, bacteriology, mortality, and duration of hospitalization at Boston City Hospital during 12 selected years between 1935 and 1972. J Infect Dis 1978; 138: 829.

3. Klatersky J. The use of synergistic combinations of antibiotics in patients with hematological diseases. Clin Haematol 1976; 5:361.

4. McLaughlin JE, Reeves DS. Clinical and laboratory evidence for inactivation of gentamicin by carbenicillin. Lancet 1971; 1:261.

5. Marks MI, Eickhoff TC. Carbenicillin: A clinical and laboratory evaluation. Ann Intern Med 1970; 73:179.

CASE 68

HISTORY

A 3-year-old boy was admitted to the hospital because of the recent onset of irritability and weakness in his right arm and leg. He had been treated a month earlier for ascariasis with thiabendazole. His father added that the child chronically ate dirt.

EXAMINATION

Physical examination revealed a boy small for his age. Temperature of 102°F. He maintained a right conjugate deviation of his eyes when not distracted. There was weakness of his right arm and leg and knee clonus.

LABORATORY DATA

The WBC count was 13,800 with 42% polys, 30% lymphs, and 16% eosinophils. A CT scan of the head showed frontal and biparietal low density lesions.

QUESTIONS

1. APPROPRIATE MANAGEMENT AT THIS POINT WOULD INCLUDE
   - A. lumbar puncture
   - B. blood cultures
   - C. craniotomy
   - D. stool exam for ova and parasites
   - E. penicillin and chloramphenicol

2. A BRAIN BIOPSY IS SHOWN IN FIGURE 3. PROPER ANTIMICROBIC DRUGS ARE
   - A. penicillin and chloramphenicol
   - B. pyrimethamine, sulfadiazene and folinic acid
   - C. thiabendazole
   - D. amphotericin B
   - E. streptomycin

The patient's toxoplasma IgM immunofluorescent antibody (IFA) titer was 1/1200; IgG IFA was 1/2400.

3. WHICH OF THE FOLLOWING SYNDROMES ARE CAUSED BY TOXOPLASMOSIS?
   - A. Chorioretinitis
   - B. Infectious mononucleosis-like illness
   - C. Encephalitis
   - D. Congenital infection with neurologic sequelae
   - E. Myocarditis

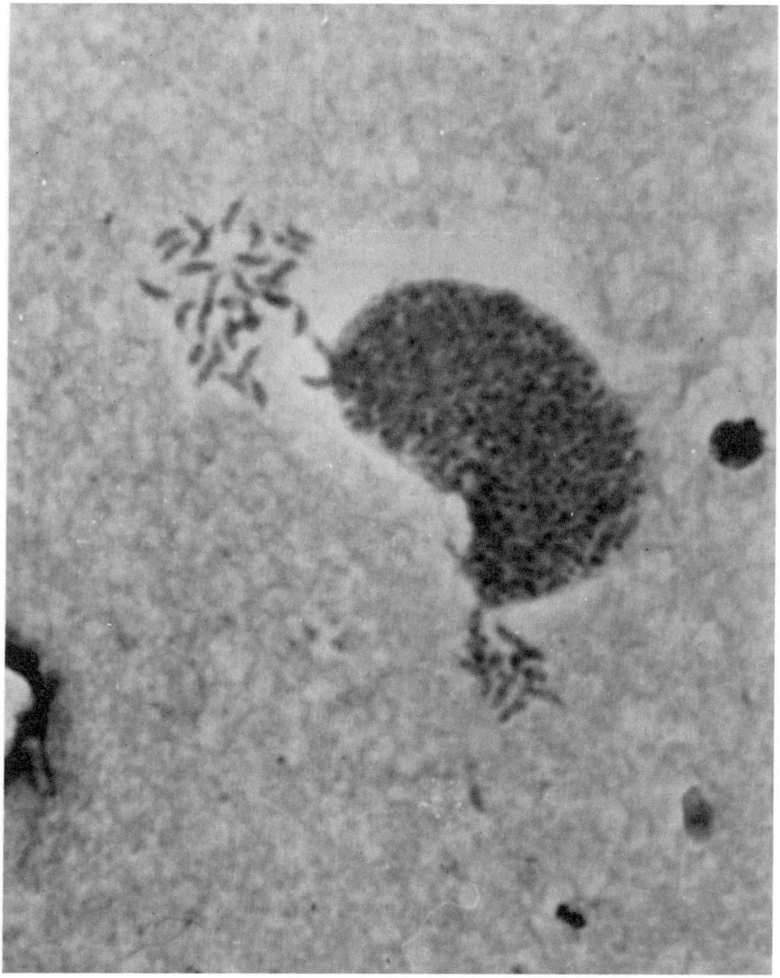

Figure 3

ANSWERS

1. (B, C, D, E) Lumbar puncture was avoided because of the risk of herniation. Stool examination was negative - no ascaris worms or eggs were seen. Penicillin and chloramphenicol were started to treat suspected bacterial brain abscess.

2. (B) Pyrimethamine and sulfadiazene have been used with some success to treat cerebral toxoplasmosis. When used together, especially in children, folinic acid must be used to prevent megaloblastic changes in the bone marrow.

3. (A, B, C, D, E) One-fourth of all cases of granulomatous uveitis are due to toxoplasmasis. In immunocompromised hosts encephalitis, myocarditis, and pneumonitis are the most common clinical manifestations. Toxoplasmosis is an important cause of congenital CNS infection.

REFERENCES

1. Symposium on toxoplasmosis. Bull NY Acad Sci 1974; 50: 107.

2. Anderson SE, Remington JS. The diagnosis of toxoplasmosis. South Med J 1975; 68:1433.

3. Mahmoud AAF, Warren KS. Algorithms in the diagnosis and management of exotic diseases. XX. Toxoplasmosis. J Infect Dis 1977; 135:493.

4. Townsend JJ, Wolinsky JS, Baringer JR, et al. Acquired toxoplasmosis. Arch Neurol 1975; 32:335.

5. Ruskin J, Remington JS. Toxoplasmosis in the compromised host. Ann Intern Med 1976; 84:193.

CASE 69

HISTORY

A 23-year-old black man was admitted to University Hospital because of bacteremia. Seven years previously he had developed symptoms and signs of the nephrotic syndrome and this necessitated initiation of chronic hemodialysis three years prior to admission. A Scribner shunt was employed. Two months before admission he noticed the onset of fever and chills during a period of home dialysis. His subsequent course is demonstrated in Figure 4. Multiple blood cultures were positive for *Bacillus alvei* during May and July. The shunt was removed in late July and one additional blood culture was positive for the same microorganism 6 days later.

QUESTIONS

1. WHICH OF THE FOLLOWING STATEMENTS REGARDING SHUNT INFECTIONS IN PATIENTS WITH CHRONIC RENAL FAILURE IS/ARE TRUE?
   - A. Staphylococci are responsible for the majority of infections in these patients
   - B. Scribner shunts are more prone to infection than Brescia fistulae or bovine heterografts
   - C. Metastatic infection is more likely to occur when *Staphylococcus aureus* is the etiologic microorganism

2. WHICH OF THE FOLLOWING STATEMENTS REGARDING INFECTIVE ENDOCARDITIS IN PATIENTS WITH A-V FISTULAE IS/ARE TRUE?
   - A. Experimental work supports the impression that an A-V fistula produces circulatory stress resulting in an endocardial surface more susceptible to bacterial localization following transient bacteremia
   - B. The most common cause of infective endocarditis in patients with maintenance hemodialysis shunts is viridans streptococcus
   - C. In patients who are receiving chronic hemodialysis vancomycin levels persist for a long duration following a single dose
   - D. Vancomycin is effective therapy for infective endocarditis caused by many gram-positive organisms
   - E. A serum bactericidial titer of 1:8 is generally adequate to assure therapeutic success in the management of infective endocarditis assuming the duration of treatment is sufficient

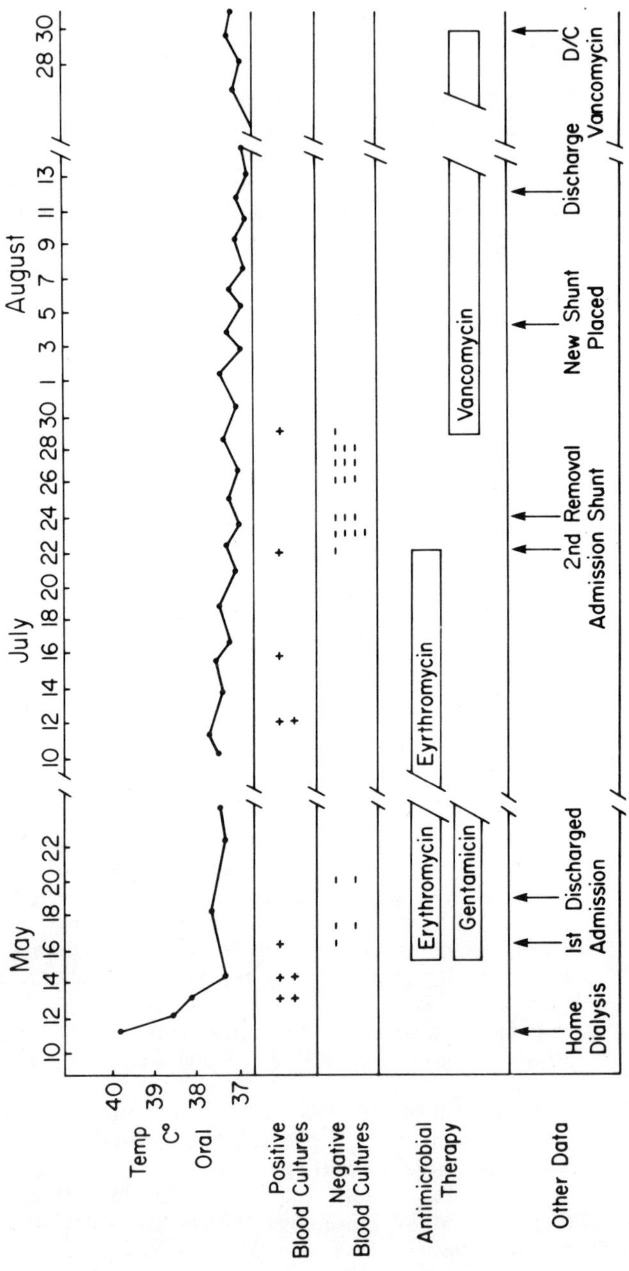
Temp
C°
Oral
40
39
38
37
Positive
Blood Cultures
Negative
Blood Cultures
Antimicrobial
Therapy
Other Data
May
July
August
Erythromycin
Gentamicin
Eyrthromycin
Vancomycin
Home
Dialysis
1st
Admission
Discharged
2nd
Admission
Removal
Shunt
New Shunt
Placed
Discharge
D/C
Vancomycin

Figure 4

3. WHICH OF THE FOLLOWING STATEMENTS REGARDING THE GENUS BACILLUS IS/ARE TRUE?

   A. Members of the genus Bacillus are aerobic, spore forming, gram-positive, rod shaped bacteria
   B. Bacteremia caused by non-anthracis bacillus strains have generally been reported from patients with serious underlying disease, intravascular foreign bodies, or both
   C. Bacillus subtilis is a recognized pathogen in the setting of endopthalmitis following trauma

ANSWERS

1. (A, B, C) Approximately two thirds of shunt infection patients undergoing chronic hemodialysis are caused by staphylococci. Staphylococcus aureus is more common than Staphylococcus epidermidis in this situation. Gram-negative aerobic bacilli are probably next most important as causes of local disease. Most all studies have shown Scribner shunts more likely to become infected than the Brescia fistulae or bovine heterografts. Staphylococcal bacteremia is more likely to result in metastatic localization in such sites as the lung, heart, brain, kidney, and joints than infection by less virulent microorganisms.

2. (A, B, C, D, E) A nice review article by Cross and Steigbigel, describes observations regarding pathogenesis of infective endocarditis in patients with A-V fistulae. It has been known for many years that experimental animals with A-V fistulae are more susceptible to infective endocarditis and the pathogenesis of endocarditis in patients with A-V fistulae appears to relate to underlying valve damage and transient bacteremia. It is not surprising that viridans streptococci are responsible for a significant proportion of infective endocarditis in patients from this population. The pharmacology of vancomycin is peculiar, following a single intravenous dose in patients with renal failure serum levels may persist 7-10 days. Vancomycin is a bactericidal drug which is active against most strains of Staphylococcus aureus, Staphylococcus epidermidis, as well as streptococci of all groups, including group D. It has been used with some success by physicians caring for patients with chronic renal failure and staphylococcal infection. In this instance it may be administered on a weekly basis. Serum levels should be checked, however, to insure sufficient activity against the infecting microorganism. For therapy of intravascular infection it is useful to confirm the adequacy of antimicrobial therapy by testing the bactericidal activity of serum obtained from the patient following a dosage of the particular drug. If the serum kills in a 1:8 dilution in vitro it is more likely that therapeutic success will follow.

3. (A, B, C) All are correct.

REFERENCES

1. Dobkin JF, Miller MH, Steigbigel NH. Septicemia in patients on chronic hemodialysis. Ann Int Med 1978; 88:28.

2. Nsouli KA, Lazarus JM, Schoenbaum SC, et al. Bacteremic infection in hemodialysis. Arch Intern Med 1979; 139: 1255.

3. Goodman JS, Crews HD, Ginn HE, Koenig MG. Medical Intelligence: Bacterial endocarditis as a possible complication of chronic hemodialysis. New Engl J Med 1969; 280:876.

4. Curtis JR, Wing AJ, Coleman JC. Bacillus cereus Bacteremia: A complication of intermittent hemodialysis. Lancet 1967; 1:136.

5. Lindholm DD, Murray JS. Persistence of vancomycin in the blood during renal failure and its treatment by hemodialysis. N Engl J Med 1966; 274:1047.

6. Eykyn S, Philip I, Evans J. Vancomycin for staphylococcal shunt infections in patients on regular hemodialysis. Brit Med J 1970; 3:80.

7. Cross AS, Steigbigel RT. Infective endocarditis and access site infections in patients on hemodialysis. Medicine 1976; 55:453.

CASE 70

HISTORY

A 12-year-old boy presents because of sore throat and fever of two days' duration. He denies any other symptoms. Physical examination reveals a pulse rate of 110 and a temperature of 103°F. The pharynx is red; both tonsils are swollen and red and are covered by a whitish exudate. There is striking anterior cervical adenopathy. The remainder of the examination is normal.

QUESTIONS

1. WHICH OF THE FOLLOWING DIAGNOSES CAN BE EXCLUDED?
   A. Streptococcal pharyngitis
   B. Infectious mononucleosis
   C. Pneumococcal pharyngitis
   D. Staphylococcal pharyngitis
   E. Adenovirus pharyngitis

2. THROAT CULTURE REVEALS MANY COLONIES OF GROUP A STREPTOCOCCI. WHICH OF THE FOLLOWING TREATMENT PROGRAMS SHOULD NOT BE EMPLOYED?
   A. Penicillin G, 250,000 units orally q.i.d. for 10 days
   B. One injection of 600,000 units of benzathine penicillin
   C. Erythromycin 1 gram/day orally for 10 days
   D. Tetracycline 1 gram/day orally for 10 days
   E. A sulfonamide 2 grams/day orally for 10 days

3. WHICH OF THE FOLLOWING IS/ARE TRUE?
   A. The symptomatic course of streptococcal pharyngitis is markedly shortened by appropriate antimicrobial therapy
   B. The incidence of subsequent rheumatic fever is definitely decreased by appropriate antimicrobial therapy of streptococcal pharyngitis
   C. The incidence of subsequent acute glomerulonephritis is definitely decreased by appropriate antimicrobial therapy of streptococcal pharyngitis
   D. Tonsillectomy is useful in preventing recurrent streptococcal pharyngitis
   E. Patients with rheumatic valvular heart disease should remain on anti-streptococcal (group A) prophylaxis for life
   F. Ingestion of food contaminated by group A streptococci may cause pharyngitis

ANSWERS

1. (C, D) Streptococcal pharyngitis, viral pharyngitis and infectious mononucleosis cannot be clinically distinguished from one another. Pneumococcus and Staphylococcus aureus do not cause pharyngitis unless there is some local or systemic host defense disorder.

2. (D, E) Approximately 20% of strains of group A streptococci are resistant to tetracycline, so this agent is not acceptable therapy for streptococcal pharyngitis unless susceptibility has been demonstrated by in vitro testing. Sulfonamides, while useful in rheumatic fever prophylaxis, are not acceptable therapy for streptococcal pharyngitis, for they fail to eradicate the organism from the pharynx and therefore do not lower the incidence of subsequent rheumatic fever.

3. (B, E, F) Specific antimicrobial therapy may shorten the course of streptococcal pharyngitis by 12-24 hours but does not markedly influence the clinical course. The incidence of rheumatic fever, but not of glomerulonephritis, is decreased by proper antimicrobial therapy of streptococcal pharyngitis. Streptococcal pharyngitis may follow ingestion of contaminated food.

REFERENCES

1. Gill FA, Hook EW. Changing patterns of bacterial resistance to antimicrobial drugs. Am J Med 1965; 39:780.

2. Hill HR, Zimmerman RA, Reid GVK, et al. Food-borne epidemic of streptococcal pharyngitis at the United States Air Force Academy. New Engl J Med 1969; 280:917.

3. Duma RJ, Weinberg AN, Medrek TF, Kunz LJ. Streptococcal infections: a bacteriologic and clinical study of streptococcal bacteremia. Medicine 1969; 48:87.

4. Wannamaker LW. Differences between streptococcal infections of the throat and of the skin. New Engl J Med 1970; 282:23.

5. Bisno AL, Pearce IA, Wall HP, et al. Contrasting epidemiology of acute rheumatic fever and acute glomerulonephritis: Nature of antecedent streptococcal infection. New Engl J Med 1970; 283:561.

CASE 71

HISTORY

A 34-year-old white man was admitted to University Hospital because of a three year history of hemoptysis, a 20 lb weight loss in the last four months, and an abnormal chest roentgenogram.

QUESTIONS

1. WHICH OF THE FOLLOWING STATEMENTS REGARDING THE DISORDER APPARENT ON X-RAY (FIGURE 5) ARE TRUE?
   - A. The infecting microorganism probably is a fungus
   - B. Invasion of lung tissue is characteristic in this disorder
   - C. Hemoptysis is common
   - D. Serologic studies are available for aid in diagnosis
   - E. Sputum cultures rarely reveal the etiologic agent

Because of recurrent hemoptysis the patient was taken to the operating room where the left upper lobe was resected. Pathologic examination revealed a cavity filled by a large fungus ball. Microscopically the fungus had the appearance of acute angle branching septate hyphae.

2. WHICH OF THE FOLLOWING STATEMENTS REGARDING ASPERGILLUS DISEASE IS/ARE TRUE?
   - A. Aspergillus may cause disseminated disease in patients with severe disorders of host defenses, such as renal transplant recipients who are receiving azothiaprine and corticosteroids
   - B. Colonization of the anterior nares sometimes anticipates more serious disease
   - C. Asperigillus fumigatus is quite susceptible to anti-fungal agents especially amphotericin B
   - D. When Asperigillus fumigatus is responsible for prosthetic heart valve endocarditis, blood cultures are rarely positive
   - E. Outbreaks of aspergillus disease have been reported in hospitals following construction projects which have stirred up dust

ANSWERS

1. (A, C, D) This case summary describes a patient with aspergillus fungus ball. Pulmonary cavities of patients with a variety of chronic destructive lung processes such as sarcoidosis, pneumoconiosis and tuberculosis may become colonized by

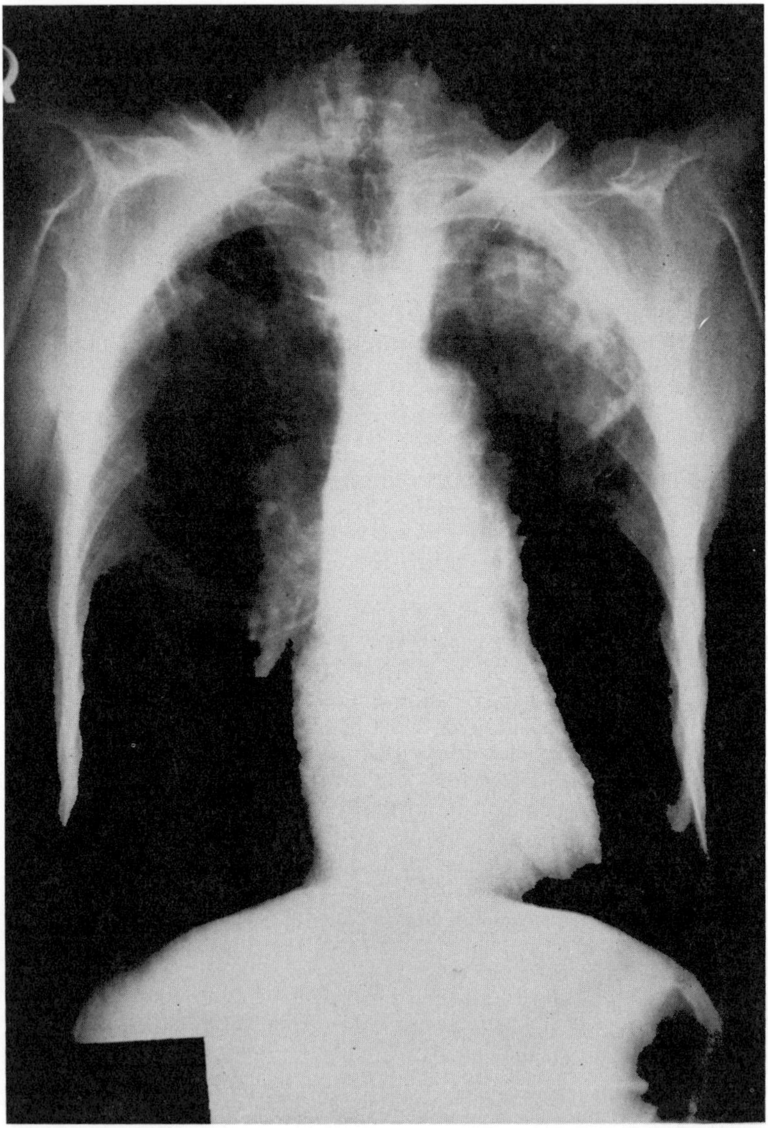

Figure 5

conidia of Aspergillus fumigatus. The fungus grows on the wall of the lesion and then peels off to partially or completely fill the cavities. The chest roentgenogram will sometimes show a characteristic air halo around a mass lesion inside a cavity. Invasion of lung tissue is unusual in this variety of aspergillus disease and the fungus ball exists in a saprophytic state frequently without causing any symptoms. Probably the most common serious complication is hemoptysis. IgG antibody to aspergillus is frequently present in the serum of patients with fungus ball and may be detected by double diffusion in agar. Sputum cultures are intermittently positive for aspergillus in patients with pulmonary fungus ball.

2. (A, B, D, E) Patients with serious disorders of host defenses against microbial invasion are susceptible to life threatening aspergillosis. Illness usually begins with fever followed in a few days by symptoms and signs of pulmonary involvement. Typically pneumonia dominates the clinical picture although metastatic disease in central nervous system, heart, and kidney may also occur. Aisner et al., report the association of nasal colonization with subsequent disease in immunosuppressed patients. While most authorities recommend amphotericin B with or without additional anti-fungal agents such as 5 flurocytosine and rifampin there is really no convincing evidence that therapy of advanced aspergillus disease in such patients is worthwhile. Occasionally when the illness is detected early or the patient's immunosuppression is reversible there may be some response to treatment. Aspergillus may cause prosthetic valve infection and this variety of endocarditis is particularly difficult to manage. Blood cultures are rarely positive. Optimal therapy probably includes early removal of the infected prosthetic device along with parenteral amphotericin therapy. The report by Arnow et al., describes an outbreak of pulmonary aspergillosis during hospital renovation. Similar epidemics have occurred in other medical centers.

REFERENCES

1. Bennett JE. Aspergillus species. In: Mandell GL, Douglas RG Jr, and Bennett JE, eds. Principles and Practices of Infectious Diseases. New York: John Wiley & Sons, 1979; 2002-08.

2. Anonymous. Aspergilloma. Lancet 1977; 1:637.

3. Aisner J, Murillo J, Schimpff S, Steere A. Invasive aspergillosis in acute leukemia: Correlation with nose culture and antibiotic use. Ann Intern Med 1979; 90:4.

4. Codish SD, Tobias JS, Hannigan M. Combined amphotericin B-flucytosine therapy in Aspergillus pneumonia. J Am Med Assn 1979; 241:2418.

5. Arnow PM, Anderson RL, Mainous D, Smith EJ. Pulmonary aspergillosis during hospital renovation. Am Rev Resp Dis 1978; 118:49.

CASE 72

HISTORY

A private physician requested Infectious Disease consultation for a patient with respiratory distress. The patient was a 63-year-old white male previously in good health except for mild chronic obstructive pulmonary disease caused by occupational exposure to coal mining and cigarette smoking. One week previously his son had returned from overseas with an illness characterized by coryza, myalgias, fever, and cough. Four days later (two days prior to admission) the patient noted the onset of a similar illness. One day prior to admission the patient's symptoms worsened with high fever, non-productive cough and mild dyspnea. On the day of admission the dyspnea became markedly worse and the patient sought medical help.

EXAMINATION

Physical examination by the private physician and the Infectious Diseases consultant revealed a seriously ill man with temperature of 104°F, tachypnea and tachycardia. Examination of the lungs revealed bilateral, diffuse, moist, medium rales on inspiration. The patient appeared mildly cyanotic; hypoxemia was confirmed by arterial blood gases which revealed a PO_2 of 45 mm on room air; pCO_2 was 23 mm. Chest roentgenogram revealed a pulmonary edema-like pattern.

QUESTIONS

1. THIS ILLNESS IS MOST CHARACTERISTIC OF
   A. pneumococcal pneumonia
   B. haemophilus influenzae pneumonia
   C. influenza virus pneumonia
   D. multiple pulmonary emboli
   E. acute myocardial infarction with acute pulmonary edema

2. WHICH OF THE FOLLOWING THERAPEUTIC MODALITIES HAVE PROVEN USEFUL IN TREATMENT OF INFLUENZA VIRUS PNEUMONIA?
   A. Corticosteroids
   B. Amantadine
   C. Lasix
   D. "Prophylactic" antimicrobial agents directed against possible superinfecting bacteria
   E. Pooled gamma globulin

3. WHICH OF THE FOLLOWING STATEMENTS REGARDING INFLUENZA VIRUS IS/ARE TRUE?

A. Russian flu (A/USSR/77, A/Brazil/78) appears to be caused by an agent which is very similar to the H1N1 strain prevalent to the United States during the 1940's and early 1950's
B. The swine flu agent represents a previously unknown mutant designated H_3N_3
C. Immunization against influenza with killed viral preparations affords solid long lasting immunity against influenza viral types included in the vaccine
D. Immunization with killed swine flu agent was associated with an increased frequency of Guillain Barre syndrome
E. In contrast to influenza A viruses influenza B viruses remain antigenically stable

ANSWERS

1. (C) Pneumonia occurring in a patient whose initial symptoms suggest uncomplicated influenza may be due to bacterial pneumonia complicating influenza, the primary influenza pneumonia syndrome, atypical pneumonia caused by the influenza virus or a mixture of influenza pneumonia and bacterial pneumonia. Primary influenza pneumonia is a serious disorder characterized by alveolitis with physical examination and roentgenologic appearance of acute pulmonary edema. It generally occurs during the first few days of influenza and the patient describes a progressively worsening disease as noted in this protocol. In contrast, bacterial pneumonia complicating influenza often appears at a time when the patient has begun to feel better. All of the choices are possible causes of his illness, but influenza virus pneumonia is the best.

2. (B, C) Amantadine and Lasix are probably useful in management of primary influenza virus pneumonia, the former because of its interference with attachment of influenza virus to host cells, and the latter because it may non-specifically improve pulmonary function in patients with severe alveolitis. Corticosteroids are of no demonstrated benefit in this syndrome; neither are prophylactic antimicrobial agents, influenza vaccine, or pooled gamma globulin.

3. (A, D) The agent responsible for the "Russian flu" of 1977-79 is classified as an H1N1 strain; it is quite similar to the virus present during the 1940's and 1950's. For this reason the groups most susceptible include children and young adults under 25 and persons older than 50, the former because they had never had experience with the virus previously and the

latter because their initial exposure to the virus had been to the H_0N_1 agent and antibody levels against H_1N_1 were low. The so-called swine flu strain of influenza A virus, isolated in 1976 and designated $H_{sw}N_1$, was believed to be similar to the agent responsible for the epidemic of 1919. Although immunization with killed influenza viral preparations is recommended, immunity so induced is marginal and of short duration. A number of studies are underway to try and develop a better preparation. There was significant increase in the Guillain Barre syndrome following the national immunization program with the swine flu strain. Recently some strains of influenza B virus have appeared with antigenic heterogeneity.

REFERENCES

1. Knight V. Influenza. In: Isselbacher KJ, Adams RD, Braunwald E, et al. Harrison's Principles and Internal Medicine. New York: McGraw-Hill Book Company, 9th Edition. 1980; 785-789.

2. Douglas RG Jr. Influenza: The disease and its complications. Hospital Practice 1976; December; 43.

3. National Influenza Immunization Program; Viral Diseases Division Bureau of Epidemiology, CDC. Follow-up on Guillain-Barre syndrome. Morbidity and Mortality Weekly Report 1977; January 7:430.

4. Antigenic analysis of Influenza B viruses. Morbidity and Mortality World Report 1980; February 8:57.

CASE 73

HISTORY

A 20-year-old basic trainee on leave from a Naval training station in the northern United States presents to the emergency room in January because of fever and backache. He was perfectly well until the day of admission when he awakened with fever, malaise and lumbar backache, all of which gradually worsened over the ensuing six hours.

EXAMINATION

Physical examination reveals an acutely ill man whose blood pressure is 105/65, pulse rate 120 and temperature 104°F. There are a few small petechiae on the volar surfaces of each forearm. The muscles of the back, arms and legs are tender to palpation. The remainder of the examination is normal.

LABORATORY DATA

Lumbar puncture reveals normal cerebrospinal fluid. Blood cultures are obtained.

QUESTIONS

1. THE APPROPRIATE COURSE OF ACTION NOW IS
   - A. discharge the patient with instructions to take aspirin
   - B. close observation
   - C. initiate treatment with twenty million units of penicillin intravenously per day
   - D. initiate treatment with twenty million units of penicillin plus 240 mg of gentamicin per day
   - E. initiate treatment with chloramphenicol, 4-6 gm per day
   - F. begin chloroquine

2. ALL BLOOD CULTURES REVEAL <u>NEISSERIA MENINGITIDIS</u>, GROUP B, RESISTANT TO SULFONAMIDES, SUSCEPTIBLE TO PENICILLIN. THE EMERGENCY ROOM STAFF WHO INITIALLY CARED FOR THE PATIENT SHOULD BE ADVISED TO
   - A. take a sulfonamide for two days
   - B. take minocycline for five days
   - C. take penicillin for five days
   - D. take rifampin for five days

3. WHICH OF THE FOLLOWING IS/ARE TRUE?
   - A. Most strains of meningococci which cause disease now are resistant to sulfonamides

B. Children frequently harbor non-pathogenic meningococci in the nasopharynx. Antibodies formed to these strains cross-react with pathogenic strains and prevent meningococcal disease when the subject is later exposed to pathogenic strains
C. It has been demonstrated in military recruits that the presence of adenovirus in the pharynx facilitates invasion by meningococci
D. A higher mortality rate is observed in patients with meningococcal meningitis than in those with only meningococcemia
E. Meningococcal pneumonia is a common problem in military recruits
F. Meningococcal vaccines have proven efficacious in preventing meningococcal disease

ANSWERS

1. (C) The clinical information is sufficiently ominous to require initiation of anti-meningococcal therapy at this time. Rocky Mountain spotted fever may present a similar clinical picture; however, it does not occur in the northern United States during the winter.

2. (D) While sulfonamides are effective in eradicating the meningococcal carrier state if the microorganism is susceptible, they are of no use in sulfonamide resistant meningococcal colonization. Minocycline and rifampin have both been demonstrated to be useful under these circumstances. The reference by Guttler et al. is a study of the use of these two antimicrobial agents in this situation. Because of the high incidence of toxicity with minocycline, rifampin is the agent of choice.

3. (A, B, C, F) Patients with fulminant meningococcal bacteremia may die without evidence of meningeal involvement. Meningococcal bacteremia accompanied by hypotension and disseminated intravascular coagulation, the so-called Waterhouse-Friderichsen syndrome, is attended by a higher mortality than is meningococcal meningitis alone. At the present time group C meningococci cause the majority of disease in the United States. The paper by Artenstein et al. in the <u>New Engl J Med</u> describes their success with the production and utilization of meningococcal vaccine.

REFERENCES

1. Feldman HA. Recent developments in the therapy and control of meningococcal infections. Disease-a-Month February, 1966; 1-31.

2. Levin S, Painter MB. The treatment of acute meningococcal infection in adults: a reappraisal. Ann Intern Med 1966; 64:1049.

3. Deal WB, Sanders E. Efficacy of rifampin in treatment of meningococcal carriers. New Engl J Med 1969; 281:641.

4. Goldschneider I, Gotschlich EC, Artenstein MS. Human immunity to the meningococcus. I. The role of humoral antibodies. J Exp Med 1969; 129:1307.

5. Goldschneider I, Gotschlich EC, Artenstein MS. Human immunity to the meningococcus. II. Development of natural immunity. J Exp Med 1969; 129:1327.

6. Guttler RB, Counts GW, Avent CK, Beaty HN. Effect of rifampin and minocycline on meningococcal carrier rales. J Inf Dis 1971; 124:199.

7. Artenstein MS, Gold R, Zimmerly JG, et al. Prevention of meningococcal disease by group C polysaccharide vaccine. New Engl J Med 1970; 282:417.

CASE 74

HISTORY

An 18-year-old mentally retarded black male was transferred to University Hospital because of fever and abnormal movements. Approximately 2 weeks before he had been seen by his private physician because of fever and pain in his knees, ankles, wrists and elbows. He was treated with cephalothin and gentamicin with no response. Three days before transfer he began to develop tremors in his hands and feet.

EXAMINATION

Physical examination reveals a young black male with choreoathetoid movements in acute distress. His temperature is 102.4°F, his blood pressure is 122/84, pulse 96 reg. The lungs are clear. The first heart sound is soft. A faint systolic ejection murmur is heard at the pulmonic area. There is no pericardial rub. Both ankles, knees, elbows, shoulders and wrists are hot, swollen, and tender. There was no rash.

LABORATORY DATA

Laboratory data included WBC count of 18,000 with 72% polys, 8% band forms and 20% lymphocytes. The SGOT was slightly elevated at 56 International Units/dl. The urinalysis was normal.

QUESTIONS

1. APPROPRIATE MANAGEMENT WOULD BE
   - A. 20 million units of penicillin and 1 gm of streptomycin a day
   - B. 1.2 million units of benzyl penicillin
   - C. salicylates
   - D. corticosteroids
   - E. withhold all drugs

2. WHICH OF THE FOLLOWING IS/ARE TRUE?
   - A. Only certain serotypes of group A streptococci appear to cause acute rheumatic fever
   - B. Only certain serotypes of group A streptococci appear to cause glomerulonephritis
   - C. Rheumatic fever may follow group A streptococci infection occurring in a variety of sites such as pharynx, skin, wounds, etc.

D. Glomerulonephritis may follow group A streptococcal infection occurring in a variety of sites such as pharynx, skin, wounds, etc.
E. Some group D streptococci have been associated with subsequent development of rheumatic fever

3. WHICH OF THE FOLLOWING IS/ARE TRUE?
A. First attacks of rheumatic fever in adults are infrequently associated with carditis
B. Only half of patients with rheumatic heart disease give a history of acute rheumatic fever
C. Sulfonamides may be used as rheumatic fever prophylaxis in patients who cannot take penicillin
D. All group A streptococci produce beta-hemolysis on a sheep blood agar

ANSWERS

1. (B, C) There is insufficient evidence to warrant high-dose treatment of endocarditis. Salicylates in high dose should be tried before using steroids.

2. (B, D) It appears that pharyngeal infections with any of the more than 50 serotypes of group A streptococci may be followed by rheumatic fever, although some strains may produce acute rheumatic fever more frequently than others. On the other hand, not all strains of group A streptococci are nephritogenic. Rheumatic fever requires pharyngeal infection whereas glomerulonephritis may follow infection at a number of sites.

3. (A, B, C) Adults typically have a lower incidence of carditis with acute rheumatic fever than children do. A recent epidemic of non-hemolytic type 18 Group A streptococcus was followed by several cases of rheumatic fever.

REFERENCES

1. Feinstein AR, Spagnuola M. The clinical pattern of acute rheumatic fever. Medicine (Baltimore) 1962; 41:279.

2. Sellers TF Jr. An epidemiologic view of rheumatic fever. Prog Cardiovasc Dis 1973; 16:303.

3. Barnett AL, Terry EE, Persellin RH. Acute rheumatic fever in adults. J Am Med Assn 1975; 232:925.

4. Bisno AL, Pearce IA, Wall HP, et al. Contrasting epidemiology of acute rheumatic fever and acute glomerulonephritis. New Engl J Med 1970; 283:561.

CASE 75

HISTORY

A 41-year-old male was referred to University Hospital because of a three month illness consisting of daily low grade fever, intermittent chills and night sweats, and progressive malaise, anorexia and 10 pound weight loss. He had been treated with two different 10 day courses of tetracycline with partial remission of his symptoms during each course, and reappearance of symptoms upon discontinuation of the antibiotic. Three weeks prior to admission he had experienced a transient episode of blurred vision in his right eye. The patient had had rheumatic fever as a child. He denied any drug allergies.

EXAMINATION

On physical examination, the patient appeared chronically ill, with blood pressure 115/80 and temperature of 101°F. His teeth were carious. A single petechia was present in the left palpebral conjunctiva and the fundi were normal. Cardiac exam showed a grade 3/6 holosystolic murmur at the apex, radiating into the left axilla, a 2/6 diastolic rumble at the apex, and a third heart sound. Rales were present over both lower lungs. The spleen was palpable 3 centimeters below the left costal margin. There was no Osler's node or Janeway's lesion, and the neurologic exam was within normal limits.

QUESTIONS

1. DIAGNOSTIC STUDIES WITHIN THE FIRST 24 HOURS OF ADMISSION IN THIS PATIENT SHOULD INCLUDE
   - A. M-mode echocardiography
   - B. three sets of blood cultures
   - C. chest x-ray
   - D. examination of urinary sediment
   - E. computerized axial tomographic (CAT) scan of brain

2. THE BEST INITIAL THERAPY, PENDING RESULTS OF BLOOD CULTURES, WOULD BE PARENTERAL
   - A. nafcillin alone
   - B. cephalosporin plus an aminoglycoside
   - C. penicillin plus an aminoglycoside
   - D. nafcillin and penicillin plus an aminoglycoside
   - E. penicillin alone

3. THE MOST COMMON INDICATION FOR SURGICAL INTERVENTION IN A PATIENT WITH NATIVE VALVE STREPTOCOCCAL INFECTIVE ENDOCARDITIS IS

A. congestive heart failure which is refractory to digitalis and diuretics
B. persistent fever and positive blood cultures due to a multiply drug resistant organism
C. recurrent emboli to the central nervous system
D. purulent pericarditis secondary to extension of infection from endocardium

Viridans streptococcus is isolated from six of six blood cultures. In an in vitro tube dilution sensitivity test the organism is killed by 0.05 ug/ml of penicillin G. It is also sensitive to tetracycline.

4. WHICH OF THE FOLLOWING REGIMENS IS/ARE ACCEPTABLE FOR THE TREATMENT OF VIRIDANS STREPTOCOCCAL ENDOCARDITIS?

A. Procaine penicillin G 1.2 million units every six hours IM for four weeks plus streptomycin 1 gm IM daily for two weeks
B. Cephalothin 2 gms IV q four hours for four weeks, or vancomycin 0.5 gm IV q six hours for four weeks, in a penicillin allergic patient
C. Tetracycline 2 gms IV daily for four weeks
D. Penicillin G 10-20 million units daily, IV for four weeks
E. Penicillin VK 1 gm PO every six hours for four weeks

ANSWERS

1. (A, B, C, D) Echocardiography is indicated to assess the severity of the mitral valve lesion and the presence or absence of vegetations. Blood cultures are mandatory to establish an etiologic diagnosis of infective endocarditis. Chest x-ray is useful in assessing cardiac size and extent of pulmonary venous hypertension. Similarly, examination of urinary sediment for WBC's, RBC's, and RBC casts is helpful in determining whether or not immune-complex glomerulonephritis is present. CAT of brain is not indicated as an emergency procedure since the patient has no focal neurologic signs or symptoms. However, should CNS problems appear, CAT would be indicated at that time to look for evidence of an embolic or hemorrhagic infarction or a mycotic aneurysm.

2. (D) The history of symptoms over a three month period in a patient with fever and heart murmur strongly suggests subacute bacterial endocarditis (SBE) as the most likely diagnosis. Viridans streptococcus is the most common cause of SBE; however,

enterococcus (a Group D streptococcus) and *Staphylococcus aureus* are also important causes. Although the patient's history of partial response to tetracycline argues most persuasively for a streptococcal etiology, initial antibiotic treatment should be directed at the three most likely pathogens, and continued until the causative agent is identified by blood cultures. Accordingly, a regimen of nafcillin for *S. aureus* and penicillin plus an aminoglycoside for viridans streptococcus and enterococcus is most appropriate.

3. (A) Patients with streptococcal endocarditis usually respond to an appropriate treatment regimen with rapid defervescence and conversion of blood cultures to negative. CNS emboli only rarely occur. Although pericarditis occurs with some frequency as a complication of acute staphylococcal endocarditis, pericarditis is a very uncommon complication of streptococcal SBE. Progressive hemodynamic instability secondary to heart failure is the most common cause of death in patients with endocarditis. Fortunately, numerous studies have shown that excision of the infected valve and valve replacement together with antibiotic therapy decreases mortality.

4. (A, B, D) Bacteriostatic agents such as tetracycline, erythromycin and chloramphenicol are unacceptable for the treatment of bacterial endocarditis. Parenteral antibiotics are preferred to insure adequate serum levels of drugs. Both regimens A (intramuscular penicillin and streptomycin) and D (intravenous penicillin) are associated with very low relapse rates.

REFERENCES

1. Pelletier LL, Petersdorf RG. Infective endocarditis: A review of 125 cases from the University of Washington Hospitals, 1963-72. Medicine 1977; 56:287.

2. Garvey GJ, Neu HC. Infective endocarditis - An evolving disease: A review of endocarditis at the Columbia-Presbyterian Medical Center, 1968-73. Medicine 1978; 57:105.

3. Lowes JA, Williams G, Tabaqchali S, et al. Ten years of infective endocarditis at St. Bartholomew's Hospital: Analysis of clinical features and treatment in relation to prognosis and mortality. Lancet 1980; 1:133.

4. Pruitt AA, Rubin RH, Karchmer AW, et al. Neurologic complications of bacterial endocarditis. Medicine 1978; 57:329.

5. Sande MA, Scheld WM. Combination antibiotic therapy of bacterial endocarditis. Ann Intern Med 1980; 92:390.

6. Karchmer AW, Moellering RC, Maki DG, et al. Single-antibiotic therapy for streptococcal endocarditis. J Am Med Assn 1979; 241:1801.

7. Richardson JV, Karp RB, Kirklin JW, Dismukes WE. Treatment of infective endocarditis: A 10 year comparative analysis. Circulation 1978; 58:589.

8. Wilson WR, Danielson GK, Giuliani ER, et al. Cardiac valve replacement in congestive heart failure due to infective endocarditis. Mayo Clin Proc 1979; 54:223.

CASE 76

HISTORY

This 28-year-old woman was admitted to University Hospital because of joint pain. Four days prior to admission she noticed the onset of swelling and discomfort in the right shoulder, followed in two days by the same symptom and sign in the right wrist. Nausea, chills, fever and night sweats began 2 days later and continued up until the time of admission. One week previously she had noted the onset of a whitish, nonpruritic vaginal discharge. There was no prior history of joint symptoms and no history of penicillin allergy.

EXAMINATION

On physical examination, she was an obese woman with a temperature of 101°F orally. The significant findings were confined to the musculoskeletal system, there was redness and swelling of the right wrist and extensor tendon sheaths of the right hand. Arthrocentesis revealed 0.5 ml of yellow, grumous material which contained numerous polymorphonuclear leukocytes but no discernable bacteria. The exudate was sent for culture.

QUESTIONS

1. INITIAL DIAGNOSTIC MANEUVERS SHOULD INCLUDE
   A. stat sedimentation rate
   B. blood culture
   C. determination of the patient's HLA type
   D. repeat physical examination looking for skin lesions

2. AT THIS POINT THERAPY SHOULD INCLUDE
   A. cephalothin and gentamicin
   B. penicillin alone
   C. tetracycline alone
   D. colchicine
   E. corticosteroids
   F. cefoxitin

Blood cultures revealed <u>Neisseria gonorrhoeae.</u>

3. WHICH OF THE FOLLOWING STATEMENTS REGARDING DISSEMINATED GONOCOCCAL INFECTION IS/ARE TRUE?
   A. More than one pathogenetic mechanism may be operative, i.e., direct microbial invasion and immune complex injury

B. Failure of putative gonococcal arthritis to improve rapidly within a few days after initiation of penicillin therapy makes that diagnosis very unlikely
C. Oral therapy may be used for treatment of gonococcal arthritis
D. Spectinomycin may be used for therapy in patients with penicillinase producing Neisseria gonorrhoeae (PPNG).

ANSWERS

1. (B, D) This case summary describes a patient with gonococcal arthritis. The disorder is generally a result of bacteremic spread from a genital site. It appears that the strains of Neisseria gonorrhoeae which cause disseminated disease are 1) more susceptible to penicillin G, 2) require arginine, hypoxanthine and uracil ($Arg^-Hxy^-Ura^-$), and 3) are more likely to cause asymptomatic genital infection than strains which do not. Blood cultures are appropriate in such patients as is careful examination of the skin for lesions of disseminated gonococcal infection. Typically these begin as erythematous macules which pustulate and may go on to hemorrhagic bulli with central necrosis. They are most commonly located on the wrists and ankles and rarely exceed 20-30 in number except in pregnant patients where they may be more numerous. A stat sedimentation rate would be of little use. There is no presently recognized association of HLA type with propensity to disseminated gonococcal infection.

2. (B) Initial therapy for the hospitalized patient is penicillin G. Some authors recommend 10 to 20 million units of aqueous penicillin a day for the first three days. If there is a dramatic response to therapy the patient may be changed to oral ampicillin to complete 7 to 10 days of treatment. Cefoxitin may be an acceptable substitute for penicillin G for therapy of urethritis in the penicillin allergic patient or in patients with disease caused by penicillinase producing gonococci.

3. (A, B, C, D) Walker et al., describe detection of circulating immune complexes in 13 of 17 patients with disseminated gonococcal infection and it appears very likely they play a role in the pathogenesis of the syndrome. Some authors have indicated the acceptability of initial high dose oral ampicillin, for instance 3.5 grams orally together with 1 gram probenecid followed by 500 mg q 6 h for 10 days for treatment of patients with disseminated gonococcal infection who are not seriously ill. On the other hand the importance of careful followup during the first few days and the possible usefulness of arthrocentesis make it generally desirable that patients with this disorder be hospitalized. Spectinomycin is acceptable in patients with PPNG.

REFERENCES

1. Sparling PF. Neisseria gonorrhoeae. In: Mandell GL, Douglas RG Jr, and Bennett JE, eds. Principles and Practices of Infectious Diseases. New York: John Wiley & Sons, 1979; 1655-66.

2. Knapp JS, Holmes KK. Disseminated gonococcal infections caused by Neisseria gonorrhoeae with unique nutritional requirements. J Infect Dis 1975; 132:204.

3. Holmes KK, Counts GW, Beaty HN. Disseminated gonococcal infection. Ann Intern Med 1971; 74:979.

4. Walker LC, Ahlin TD, Tung KSK, et al. Circulating immune complexes in disseminated gonorrheal infection. Ann Intern Med 1978; 89:28.

5. Handsfield HH, Wiesner PJ, Holmes KK. Treatment of the gonococcal arthritis-dermatitis syndrome. Ann Intern Med 1976; 84:661.

6. U.S. Department of Health, Education, and Welfare, Public Health Service, Center for Disease Control; Atlanta, GA. Gonorrhea: Center for Disease Control recommended treatment schedules. Ann Int Med 1979; 90:809.

7. Wiesner PJ, Handsfield HH, Holmes KK. Low antibiotic resistance of gonococci causing disseminated infection. New Engl J Med 1973; 288:1221.

8. Cooke CL, Owen DS Jr, Irby R, Toone E. Gonococcal Arthritis: A survey of 54 cases. J Am Med Assn 1971; 217(2): 204.

9. Berg SW, Kilpatrick ME, Harrison WO, McCutchan JA. Cefoxitin as a single-dose treatment for urethritis caused by penicillinase-producing Neisseria gonorrhoeae. New Engl J Med 1979; 301(10):509.

10. Wiesner PJ, Thompson SE. Gonococcal Disease. Disease-A-Month 1980; 26(5):1-44.

INDEX: By Case Number